About this Series

IDEAS IN PROGRESS is a commercially published series of working papers dealing with alternatives to industrial society. It is our belief that the ills and frustrations which have overtaken mankind are not merely due to industrial civilization's inadequate planning and faulty execution, but are caused by fundamental errors in our basic thinking about goals. This series is designed to question and rethink the underlying concepts of many of our institutions and to propose alternatives. Unless this is done soon society will undoubtedly create even greater injustices and inequalities than at present. It is to correct this trend that authors are invited to submit short texts of work in progress of interest not only to their colleagues but also to the general public. The series fosters direct contact between the author and the reader. It provides the author with the opportunity to give wide circulation to his draft while he is still developing an idea. It offers the reader an opportunity to participate critically in shaping this idea before it has taken on a definitive form.

Future editions of a paper may include the author's revisions and critical reactions from the public. Readers are invited to write directly to the author of the present volume at the following address:

Ivan Illich, CIDOC, Apdo. 479, Cuernavaca, Mor., Mexico

THE PUBLISHERS

ABOUT THE AUTHOR

Ivan Illich was born in 1926. He studied theology and philosophy at the Gregorian University in Rome and obtained a doctorate in history at the University of Salzburg. He went to the United States in 1951, where he served as assistant pastor in an Irish-Puerto Rican parish in New York City. From 1956 to 1960 he was vice-rector of the Catholic University of Puerto Rico. Illich was a co-founder of the Center for Intercultural Documentation (CIDOC) in Cuernavaca, Mexico, and since 1964 he has directed research seminars on 'Institutional Alternatives in a Technological Society', with special focus on Latin America. Ivan Illich's writings have appeared in *The New York Times, The New York Review of Books, The Saturday Review, Esprit, Kursbuch, Siempre, Excelsior de Mexico, America, Commonweal, Les Temps Modernes, Le Monde, The Guardian* and *The Lancet*. He is the author of *Celebration of Awareness, Deschooling Society, Tools for Conviviality,* and *Energy and Equity*.

MEDICAL NEMESIS

IDEAS IN PROGRESS

MEDICAL NEMESIS

THE EXPROPRIATION OF HEALTH

Ivan Illich

CALDER & BOYARS

First published in Great Britain in 1975
by Calder & Boyars Ltd
18 Brewer Street, London W1

ISBN 0 7145 1095 5 Cased Edition
ISBN 0 7145 1096 3 Paperback Edition

Printed in Great Britain
by Ebenezer Baylis and Son Limited
The Trinity Press, Worcester, and London

TABLE OF CONTENTS

7

PART III STRUCTURAL IATROGENESIS

*The Devotional Dance of the Dead, page 124.
The Danse Macabre, page 126. Bourgeois Death,
page 134. Clinical Death, page 139. Trade
Union Claims to a Natural Death, page 141.
Death under Intensive Care, page 144.*

PART IV THE POLITICS OF HEALTH

*Industrialized Nemesis, page 154. Endemic
Nemesis, page 155. Medical Nemesis, page 159.
Veiled Nemesis, page 161. From Inherited
Myth to Respectful Procedure, page 161. The
Right to Health, page 165. Hygiene as a Virtue,
page 167.*

PREFACE

THIS essay is the outline for a seminar I will conduct in 1975 at CIDOC in Cuernavaca. It is also the first published version of a book which is still, despite its appearance in this form, in the process of being written. The footnotes reflect the twofold nature of the text: they document facts, but they also provide potential readers with suggestions on related issues which ought to be explored further and present the kind of bibliographical guidance I would have liked to have found when I first began as an outsider to delve into the subject of health-care.

This working paper was written for the series *Ideas in Progress*, originated by my English publisher, which provides a public channel for sharing this draft not only with colleagues but also with the general public while I am still struggling with the final formulation of my ideas.

My thinking on medical institutions was shaped over several years in periodic conversations with John McKnight and Roslyn Lindheim. McKnight is now working on a book which deals with the political process by which service institutions can be made innocuous without depriving society of their continued existence. Roslyn Lindheim, an architect, is about to publish in the *Ideas in Progress* series a critique of hospitalized space.

Jean Pierre Dupuy and Rick Carlson are two other participants in our conversations. Dupuy will shortly publish a book focusing on the medicalization of drugs in France, whereas Carlson's critique of American medicine will give considerable space to non-conventional alternatives to the prevailing medical ideology.[0]

[0] LINDHEIM, Roslyn. *The hospitalization of space.* To be published by Calder and Boyars in 1975. For partial drafts, see CIDOC DOC. I/V 74/73 and 74/74. DUPUY, Jean-Pierre, and KARSENTY, Serge. *L'invasion pharmaceutique.* To be published by Ed. du Seuil, October, 1974. CARLSON, Rick. *The end of medicine.* A draft manuscript, Santa Barbara, California, January, 1973, to be published in 1975. Reprinted in CIDOC Antologia A3.

We have read each other's manuscripts at several stages, and they will find their ideas and expressions in these pages, even when I do not explicitly quote them. Abraham and Irene Díaz González, Douglas Wright, John Bradley, André Gorz, Susan Hunt, Joseph Cunneen and Vramalingaswami have given me critical and constructive assistance. John S. Bradshaw has given generous guidance and criticism at proof stage. Only I am to blame for not having accepted all his advice.

This essay could never have been written without the collaboration of Valentina Borremans. For several years she has patiently assembled the documentation on which it is based, and refined my judgement and sobered my expression with her constant criticism. The chapter on the industrialization of death is a summary of the notes she has assembled for her own book on the face of death.

Ivan Illich
Cuernavaca
August 23, 1974

INTRODUCTION

THE medical establishment has become a major threat to health. Dependence on professional health care affects all social relations. In rich countries medical colonization has reached sickening proportions; poor countries are quickly following suit. This process, which I shall call the 'medicalization of life', deserves articulate political recognition. Medicine is about to become a prime target for political action that aims at an inversion of industrial society. Only people who have recovered the ability for mutual self-care by the application of contemporary technology will be ready to limit the industrial mode of production in other major areas as well.

A professional and physician-based health care system which has grown beyond tolerable bounds is sickening for three reasons: it must produce clinical damages which outweigh its potential benefits; it cannot but obscure the political conditions which render society unhealthy; and it tends to expropriate the power of the individual to heal himself and to shape his or her environment. The medical and para-medical monopoly over hygienic methodology and technology is a glaring example of the political misuse of scientific achievements to strengthen industrial rather than personal growth. Such medicine is but a device to convince those who are sick and tired of society that it is they who are ill, impotent and in need of technical repair. I will deal with these three levels of sickening medical impact in three sections.

The balance sheet of medical achievement will be drawn up in the first chapter. Many people are already apprehensive about medicine and only need data to substantiate their misgivings. Doctors already find it necessary to bolster their credibility by demanding that many treatments now common be formally outlawed. Restrictions on medical performance which professionals have come to consider mandatory are often so radical that they are not acceptable to the majority of politicians. The lack of effectiveness of costly and high-risk medicine is a fact from which I start, not a key issue I want to dwell on.

The second section comprises three chapters. It describes some of the social symptoms resulting from the medicalization of health, interprets them as ills typical of over-industrialized civilization, and deals with five types of political response, all futile.

The third section focuses on the expropriation of health, and the transformation of pain, impairment and death from a personal challenge into a technical problem. The final section distinguishes between two modes in which the person relates and adapts to his environment: autonomous (i.e. self-governing) coping, and heteronomous (i.e. administered) maintenance and management. It concludes by demonstrating that only a political programme aimed at the limitation of professional medicine enables people to recover their powers for health care.

PART I
CLINICAL IATROGENESIS

1 THE EPIDEMIC OF MODERN MEDICINE

THE diseases afflicting Western societies have undergone dramatic changes. In the course of a century, so many mass killers have vanished that two-thirds of all deaths are now associated with the diseases of old age.[1] Those who die young, are more often than not victims of accidents, violence and suicide.[2]

These changes in health status are generally equated with progress and are attributed to more or better medical care. In fact, there is no evidence of any direct relation between this mutation of sickness and the so-called progress of medicine.[3] In addition, an expanding proportion of the new disease burden of the last 15 years is itself the result of medical intervention in favour of

[1] Perinatal mortality must be excluded. In all European countries it exceeds all other mortality during the first 30 years of life. LONGONE, P. *Mortalité et morbidité*, in: Population et Sociétés. Bulletin Mensuel d'Informations Démographiques, Economiques, Sociales. No. 43, January, 1972.

[2] LALONDE, Marc. *A new perspective on the health of Canadians*, a working document. Government of Canada, Ottawa, April, 1974. This French-English bilingual report contains a multi-coloured centrefold documenting the change in mortality for Canada in a series of graphs. For France see: LONGONE, P. *Les maux de la richesse. Morts violentes et surmortalité masculine*, in: Population et Sociétés. Bulletin Mensuel d'Informations Démographiques, Economiques Sociales. No. 11, February, 1969, and *La surmortalité masculine*, in: Population et Sociétés. Bulletin Mensuel d'Informations Démographique, Economiques, Sociales. No. 59, 1 June, 1973, indicates that in France deaths from car accidents represent 66% of all male and 39% of all female deaths between the ages of 15 and 34, 50% of all deaths of boys 5–14 and 33% of all deaths between 1 and 4 years of age.

[3] DUBOS, René. *Mirage of health, utopias, progress and biological change*. New York, Anchor Books, 1959, was the first who effectively exposed the delusion of producing 'better health' as a dangerous and infectious medically-sponsored disease. MCKEOWN, Thomas and MCLACHLAN, Gordon, eds. *Medical history and medical care: a symposium of perspectives*, Oxford Univ. Press, 1971, introduce the sociology of medical pseudo-progress. POWLES, John, *On the limitations of modern medicine*, in: Science, Medicine and Man. Vol. 1, pp. 1–30, Great Britain, Pergamon Press, 1973, gives a critical selection of recent English-language literature to this first section of chapter I. CARLSON, see note 0, is a lawyer. His essay is 'an empirically based brief, theoretical in nature'. For his indictment of American medicine he has chosen those dimensions for which he had complete evidence of a nature he could handle. DUPUY-KARSENTY, see note 0, combines ample empirical research on the effectiveness of contemporary medicine with vast documentation.

people who are or might become sick: (1) The impotence of medical services to change life expectancy, (2) the insignificance of most contemporary clinical care in the curing of disease, (3) the magnitude of medically inflicted damage to health, and (4) the futility of medical counter-measures to sickening medical care are all obvious, well documented—and well repressed.

Doctors' Effectiveness—An Illusion

The study of the evolution of disease patterns provides evidence that during the last century doctors have affected such patterns no more profoundly than did priests during earlier times. Epidemics came and went, imprecated by both and untouched by either. They are not modified any more decisively by the rituals performed in medical clinics than by the exorcisms customary at religious shrines.[4] Discussion on the future of health care might usefully begin with this recognition.

The infections which prevailed at the outset of the industrial age can illustrate how medicine came by its reputation. Tuberculosis, for instance, reached a peak over two generations. In New York the death rate was certainly very high indeed in 1812 and declined to 370 per 10,000 by 1882 when Koch cultured and stained the first bacillus. The rate was down to 180 when the first sanatorium was opened in 1910, even though, 'consumption' still held second place in the mortality tables. After World War II, before antibiotics came into use, it had slipped into eleventh place with a rate of 48. Cholera, dysentery and typhoid similarly peaked and dwindled outside medical control. By the time their etiology was understood or their therapy had become specific, they had lost much of their relevance.[5] The combined death rate for scarlet fever, diphtheria, whooping cough and measles from 1860 to 1965 for children up to 15 shows that nearly 90% of the total decline in the death rate over this period had occurred before the introduction of antibiotics and widespread immunization

[4] DUBOS, René. *The dreams of reason, science and utopia.* N.Y., Columbia University Press, especially p. 66 and ff.
[5] DUBOS, René. *Man adapting.* New Haven, Yale Univ. Press, 1965, especially chapter 7 on the evolution of microbial diseases, and the bibliography to this chapter.

against diphtheria.[6] Part of the explanation might be a decline in the virulence of micro-organisms and improved housing, but by far the most important factor was a higher host-resistance due to improved nutrition. In poor countries today, diarrhoea and upper respiratory tract infections occur more frequently, last longer and lead to higher mortality where nutrition is low, no matter how much or little medical care is available.[7] In England, by the middle of the 19th century, infectious epidemics were replaced by major malnutrition syndromes, such as rickets and pellagra. These in turn peaked and vanished, to be replaced by the diseases of early childhood and then by duodenal ulcers in young men. When these declined, the modern epidemics took over: coronary heart disease, emphysema, bronchitis and obesity, hypertension, cancer (especially of the lung), arthritis, diabetes, and the so-called mental disorders. Despite intensive research, we have no satisfactory explanation for the genesis of these changes.[8] But two things are certain: the professional practice of physicians cannot be credited with the elimination of old forms of mortality, nor ought it to be blamed for the increased expectancy of life spent suffering from the new diseases.

Analysis of disease trends shows that the environment is the primary determinant of the state of general health of any population.[9] Food, housing, working conditions, neighbourhood cohesion, as well as the cultural mechanisms which make it possible to keep the population stable, play the decisive role in determining how healthy grown-ups feel and at what age adults tend to die. As older pathogens fade a new kind of malnutrition is becoming the most rapidly expanding modern epidemic: one

[6] PORTER, R. R. *The contribution of the biological and medical sciences to human welfare.* Presidential Address to the British Association for the Advancement of Science, Swansea Meeting, 1971. Published by the Association, p. 95, 1972.

[7] SCRIMSHAW, N. S.; TAYLOR, C. E. and GORDON, John E. *Interactions of nutrition and infection.* World Health Organization, Geneva, 1968.

[8] CASSEL, John. *Physical illness in response to stress.* 32 pages mimeo. CIDOC I/V NEM. 06.

[9] WINKELSTEIN, Warren Jr. *Epidemiological considerations underlying the allocation of health and disease care resources,* in: International Journal of Epidemiology, Vol. 1, No. 1, Oxford Univ. Press, 1972. The author points out that mid-century English doctors had already recognized the environment as a primary determinant for the health status of populations. He refers especially to E. CHADWICK, 1842, and L. SHATTUCK, 1850. See also LAVE, Lester B. and SESKIN, Eugene P. *Air pollution and human health,* in: Science, Vol. 169, No. 3947, 21 August, 1970, pp. 723–733.

third of humanity survives on a level of undernourishment which would formerly have been lethal, while more and more people absorb poisons and mutagens in their food.[10]

Some modern techniques, often developed with the contribution of doctors, and optimally effective when they become part of the environment or are applied by the general public, have determined changes in general health, but to a lesser degree. Into this category belong contraceptives and such non-medical health measures as the treatment of water or excrement, the use of soap and scissors by midwives, the smallpox vaccination of infants, and a few antibacterials and insecticides. The most recent shifts of mortality from younger to older groups can be explained by the spread of these procedures and devices.

In contrast to the natural environment and modern though non-professional health measures, the specifically medical treatment of people is nowhere and never significantly related to a decline in the compound disease burden or to a rise in life expectancy.[11] Neither the rate of doctors in a population, nor the clinical tools at their disposal, nor the number of hospital beds are causal factors in the striking changes in overall patterns of disease. The new techniques available to recognize and treat such conditions as pernicious anaemia and hypertension, or to correct

[10] So far, world hunger and world malnutrition have increased with industrial development. SAHLINS, Marshall. *Stone age economics*. Chicago, Aldine-Atherton, 1972, p. 23. ... 'one third to one half of humanity are said to be going to bed hungry every night. In the Stone Age the fraction must have been much smaller. This is the era of unprecedented hunger. Now, in the time of the greatest technical power, starvation is an institution.' DAVIS, Adelle. *Let's eat right to keep fit*. Rev. and updated ed., N.Y., Harcourt Brace, 1970, a well-documented report on the qualitative decline of the U.S. diet with the rise of industrialization, and the reflections of this decline in U.S. health. HARMER, Ruth Mulvey, *Unfit for human consumption*, Prentice Hall, N.J., 1971, claims that the World Health Organization has a vested interest in the continued use of poisonous pesticides because of its public health programmes. WELLFORD, Harrison. *Sowing the wind*. A report for Ralph Nader's Center for the Study of Responsive Law on food safety and the chemical harvest. Introduction by Ralph Nader. New York, Bantam paper ed., 1973. A collaborator of Ralph Nader reports on pesticide concentration in common foods. The misuse of pesticides threatens the farmer even more than the city dweller: it destroys his health, raises the cost of production and tends to lower long-term yields.

[11] STEWART, Charles T. Jr. *Allocation of resources to health*, in: The Journal of Human Resources, VI, 1, 1971 classifies resources devoted to health as treatment, prevention, information and research. In all nations of the Western hemisphere, prevention (potable water) and education are significantly related to life-expectancy, but none of the 'treatment variables' are so related.

18

congenital malformations by surgical interventions, redefine but do not reduce morbidity. The fact that there are more doctors where certain diseases have become rare has little to do with their ability to control or eliminate them.[12] It simply means that doctors deploy themselves as they like, more so than other professionals, and that they tend to gather where the climate is healthy, where the water is clean, and where people work and can pay for their services.

Useless Medical Treatment

Awe-inspiring medical technology has combined with egalitarian rhetoric to create the dangerous delusion that contemporary medicine is highly effective. Although contemporary medical practice is built on this erroneous assumption, it is contradicted by informed medical opinion.[13]

During the last generation, a limited number of specific procedures have indeed become effective. Those which are applicable to widespread diseases are usually very inexpensive: unless they are monopolized for personal use, they require a minimum of personal skills, materials or hotel services from hospitals. In contrast, most of the skyrocketing medical expenditures are destined for diagnosis and treatment of no or of doubtful effectiveness. This can best be illustrated by distinguishing between infectious and non-infectious diseases.

Chemotherapy has played a significant role in the control of pneumonia, gonorrhoea and syphilis. Death from pneumonia, once the 'old man's friend', declined yearly by 5 to 8% after sulphonamides and antibiotics came on the market. Malaria, typhoid, syphilis and yaws can be cured quite easily. The rising

[12] STALLONES, Reuel A. *Environnement, écologie et épidémologie* (texte abrégé de la quatrième conférence du Cycle de Conférences Scientifiques OPS/OMS, Washington, 30 September 1971). Shows that there is a strong positive correlation in the USA between a high rate of doctors in the general population and high coronary disease, while the correlation is strongly negative for cerebral vascular disease. He points out that this says nothing about a possible influence doctors may have on either. Morbidity and mortality are an integral part of the human environment and unrelated to the efforts made to control any specific disease.

[13] The model study on this matter at present seems to be COCHRANE, A. L. *Effectiveness and efficiency: random reflections on health services.* The Nuffield Provincial Hospitals Trust, 1972. See also British Medical Journal, 1974, vol. 4, p. 5.

rate of venereal disease is due to new mores, not to bad medicine. The reappearance of malaria is due to the development of pesticide-resistant mosquitoes and not to any lack of new anti-malarial drugs. Immunization has almost wiped out paralytic poliomyelitis, a disease of developed countries. Vaccines have made some contribution to the decline of whooping cough and measles. Certainly, at least for the moment, the medical impact on these infections confirms the popular belief of 'progress in medicine'. But for *most* other infections, medicine can show no comparable results. Drug treatment did reduce mortality from tuberculosis, tetanus, diphtheria and scarlet fever, but in the total decline of mortality or morbidity from these diseases, chemotherapy played a minor, possibly insignificant role. Malaria, leishmaniasis and sleeping sickness have receded for a time under the onslaught of chemical attacks, but are now on the rebound.[14]

The effectiveness of medical intervention in combating non-infectious diseases is even more questionable. Effective progress has indeed been demonstrated in a few conditions: the partial prevention of caries through fluoridation of water is possible, though at a cost not fully understood. Replacement therapy lessens the direct impact of diabetes, but only in the short run. As a result of intravenous feeding, blood transfusions and oxygen tents,[15] more people survive trauma. The diagnostic value of the Papanicolaou vaginal smear test has been proven, and if the tests are given often enough, early intervention for cervical cancer increases the five-year survival rate. Skin cancer treatment is highly effective. We lack clear evidence for effective treatment of all other cancers.[16] Breast cancer is the most common form. The five-year survival rate is 50% no matter with what frequency medical check-ups are performed and no matter what

[14] See note 47.

[15] UNIVERSITIES GROUP DIABETES PROGRAM. *A study of the effects of hypoglycemic agents on vascular complications in patients with adult onset diabetes. II. Mortality results, 1970,* in: Diabetes, 19, suppl. 2. KNATTERUD, G. L.; MEINERT, C. L.; KLIMT, C. R.; OSBORNE, R. K.; MARTIN, D. B. *Effects of hypoglycemic agents on vascular complications in patients with adult onset diabetes. 1971,* in: Journal of American Medicine Association, 217, 6, 777. COCHRANE, see note 13, comments on the last two. They suggest that giving tolbutamide and phenformin is definitely disadvantageous in the treatment of mature diabetics and that there is no advantage in giving insulin rather than a diet.

[16] MCKINNON, N. E. *The effects of control programs on cancer mortality,* in: Canadian Medical Association Journal, 82, June 25, 1960, pp. 1308–1312.

treatment is used.[17] It has not been shown that this rate differs from that of untreated cancer.[18] Although practising doctors tend to stress the importance of early detection and treatment of this and several other types of cancer, epidemiologists have begun to doubt if early intervention would alter survival rates.[19]

Surgery and chemotherapy for rare congenital and rheumatic heart disease has increased the chances for an active life for some of those who suffer from these conditions.[20] The medical treatment of common cardiovascular[21] and heart disease,[22] however, is only partially effective. The drug treatment of high blood pressure is effective for the few in whom it is a malignant condition and can do serious harm to those in whom it is not.[23]

Doctor-inflicted Injuries

Unfortunately, the futility of medical care is the least of the torts a proliferating medical enterprise inflicts on society. The impact of medicine constitutes one of the most rapidly expanding epidemics of our time. The pain, dysfunction, disability and even anguish[24] which result from technical medical intervention now

[17] BREAST CANCER SYMPOSIUM. *Points in the practical management of breast cancer. 1969*, in: Breast Journal Surg. 56, 782.

[18] LEWISON, Edwin F. *An appraisal of long-term results in surgical treatment of breast cancer*, in: Journal of the American Medical Association, 186, Dec. 14, 1963. pp. 975–978.

[19] SUTHERLAND, Robert. *Cancer: the significance of delay*. London, Butterworth and Co., 1960, pp. 196–202. Also ATKINS, Hedley et al. *Treatment of early breast cancer: a report after ten years of clinical trial* in: Brit. Med. Journ. 1972, 2, pp. 423–429 also p. 417.

[20] KUTNER, Ann G. *Current status of steroid therapy in rheumatic fever*, in: American Heart Journal, 70, August, 1965, pp. 147–149. THE RHEUMATIC FEVER WORKING PARTY OF THE MEDICAL RESEARCH COUNCIL OF GREAT BRITAIN AND THE SUBCOMMITTEE OF PRINCIPAL INVESTIGATORS OF THE AMERICAN COUNCIL ON RHEUMATIC FEVER AND CONGENITAL HEART DISEASE, AMERICAN HEART ASSOCIATION, *Treatment of acute rheumatic fever in children: a cooperative clinical trial of ACTH, cortisone and aspirin*, in : British Medical Journal, 1, 1955, pp. 555–574.

[21] BREST, Albert N. *Treatment of coronary occlusive disease: critical review*, in: Diseases of the Chest, 45, January, 1964, pp. 40–45. LINDSAY, Malcolm I., SPIEKERMAN, Ralph E. *Re-evaluation of therapy of acute myocardial infarction*, in: American Heart Journal, 67, April, 1964, pp. 559–564. CAIN, Harvey D. et al. *Current therapy of cardiovascular disease*, in: Geriatrics, 18, July, 1963. pp. 507–518.

[22] MATHER, H. G.; PEARSON, N. G.; READ, K. L. et al. *Acute myocardial infarction: home and hospital treatment*, in: British Medical Journal, 1971, vol. 3, pp. 334–338.

[23] COMBINED STAFF CLINIC. *Recent advances in hypertension*, in: American Journal of Medicine, 39, Cot. 1965, pp. 634–638.

[24] SHEY, Herbert H. *Iatrogenic anxiety*, in: Psychiatric Quarterly, Vol. 45, 1971, pp. 343–56.

rival the morbidity due to traffic, work and even war-related activities. Only modern malnutrition is clearly ahead.

The technical term for the new epidemic of doctor-made disease, *Iatrogensis*, is composed of the Greek words for 'physician' (*iatros*) and for 'origins' (*genesis*). Iatrogenic disease comprises only illness which would not have come about unless sound and professionally recommended treatment had been applied.[25] Within this definition, a patient can sue his therapist if the latter, in the course of his treatment, has not applied a recommended treatment and thus risked making him sick.

In a more general and more widely accepted sense, clinical iatrogenic disease comprises all clinical conditions for which remedies, physicians or hospitals are the pathogens or 'sickening' agents. I will call this plethora of therapeutic side-effects *clinical iatrogenesis*.[26]

Medicines have always been potentially poisonous, but their unwanted side-effects have increased with their effectiveness and widespread use.[27] Every 24 to 36 hours, from 50% to 80% of adults in the U.S. and the U.K. swallow a medically prescribed chemical. Some take a wrong drug, others get a contaminated or old batch, others a counterfeit,[28] others take several drugs

---

[25] A standard textbook: MOSER, Robert H. *Diseases of medical progress: a study oj iatrogenic disease*. A contemporary analysis of illness produced by drugs and other therapeutic procedure. Foreword by ADAMS, F. Denette. Springfield, USA, Charles C. Thomas, 1969.

[26] It was already studied by the Arabs. Al-Razi was the medical chief of the hospital of Bagdad and lived A.D. 865–925. According to Al-Nadim in the Fihrist, chapter 7, section 3, he was concerned with the medical study of iatrogenesis. At the time of Al-Nadim, A.D. 935, three books and one letter on the subject were still available. 'The mistakes in the purpose of physicians', 'On purging fever patients before the time is ripe', on 'The reason why the ignorant physicians, the common people and the women in cities are more successful than men of science in treating certain diseases and on the excuses which physicians make for this', and the letter explaining 'Why a clever physician does not have the power to heal all diseases, for that is not within the realm of the possible.'

[27] DUPUY, J. P., FERRY, J., KARSENTY, S., WORMS, H. *La consommation de médicaments, approche psycho-socio-économique*. Paris, CEREBE, 1971, Rapport principal 244 pp., annexes 757 pp., mimeo.

[28] KREIG, Margaret. *Black market medicine*. N.J., Prentice-Hall, 1967. 304 pp. Reports and proves that an increasing percentage of articles sold by legitimate professional pharmacies are inert counterfeit drugs which are indistinguishable in packaging and presentation from the trade-marked product. Detection is increasingly difficult, and prosecution of the Mafia behind this black market is beyond the control of current law-enforcement agencies.

which are dangerous[29] or take them in dangerous combinations, others receive injections with improperly sterilized syringes or brittle needles. Some drugs are addictive, others mutilating, others mutagenic, although perhaps only in synergy with food colouring or insecticide.[30] In some patients, antibiotics alter the normal bacterial flora and induce a super-infection, permitting more resistant organisms to proliferate and invade the host. Other drugs contribute to the breeding of drug-resistant strains of bacteria.[31] Subtle kinds of poisoning thus have spread even faster than the bewildering variety and ubiquity of nostrums.[32] Unnecessary surgery is a standard procedure.[33] Disabling non-diseases result from the medical treatment of non-existent diseases and are on the increase: the number of children disabled

[29] MINTZ. Morton. *By prescription only.* A report on the roles of the United States Food and Drug Administration, the American Medical Association, pharmaceutical manufacturers and others in connection with the irrational and massive use of prescription drugs that may be worthless, injurious or even lethal. Boston, Houghton Mifflin, 1967. (Second ed. revised and updated, previously published under the title: *The therapeutic nightmare.*)

[30] SAX, Irving. *Dangerous properties of industrial materials.* New York, Van Nostrand, 1968. MEYLER, L. *Side effects of drugs.* Williams & Wilkins, 1972.

[31] BEATY, Harry N. and PETERSDORF, Robert G. *Iatrogenic factors in infectious disease,* in: Annals of Internal Medicine. Vol. 65, No. 4, October 1966, pp. 641–56.

[32] Every year a million people—that is, 3 to 5% of all hospital admissions—are admitted primarily because of a negative reaction to drugs. WADE, Nicholas. *Drug regulation: FDA replies to charges by economists and industry,* in: Science, 179, February 23, 1973, pp. 775–777.

[33] VAYDA, Eugene. *A comparison of surgical rates in Canada and in England and Wales,* in: The New England Journal of Medicine. Vol. 289, No. 23, Dec. 6, 1973, pp. 1224–1229. This comparison shows that surgical rates in Canada (1968) were 1·8 times greater for men and 1·6 times greater for women than in England. Discretionary operations such as tonsillectomy and adenoidectomy, hemorrhoidectomy and inguinal herniorrhaphy were two or more times higher. Cholcecystectomy rates were more than five times greater. The main determinants may be the differences in payment of health services and available hospital beds and surgeons. LEWIS, Charles E. *Variations in the incidence of surgery,* in: The New England Journal of Medicine, 281 (6): 880–884, 16th October, 1969. Reprinted in CIDOC *Antologia A8.* LEWIS finds three to fourfold variations in regional rates for six common surgical procedures in the U.S.A. The number of surgeons available was found to be the significant predictor in the incidence of surgery. See also DOYLE, James C. *Unnecessary hysterectomies.* Study of 6,248 operations in thirty-five hospitals during 1948, in: J.A.M.A., Vol. 151, No. 5, January 31, 1953. Reprinted in CIDOC *Antologia A8.* DOYLE, James C. *Unnecessary ovariectomies.* Study based on the removal of 704 normal ovaries from 546 patients, in: J.A.M.A., Vol. 148, No. 13, March 29, 1952, pp. 1105–1111. WELLER, Thomas H. *Pediatric perceptions. The pediatrician and iatric infectious disease,* in: Pediatrics, Vol. 51, No. 4, April, 1973. See also BRANDIS, C. V. *Art und Kunstfehlervorwurf.* Goldmann, Wissenschaftliches Taschenbuch, 1971.

in Massachussetts from cardiac non-disease exceeds the number of children under effective treatment for cardiac disease.[34]

Doctor-inflicted pain and infirmity have always been a part of medical practice.[35] Professional callousness, negligence and sheer incompetence are age-old forms of malpractice.[36] With the transformation of the doctor from an artisan exercising a skill on personally known individuals into a technician applying scientific rules to classes of patients, malpractice acquired a new anonymous, almost respectable status. What had formerly been considered an abuse of confidence and a moral fault can now be rationalized into the occasional breakdown of equipment and operators. In a complex technological hospital, negligence becomes 'random human error', callousness becomes 'scientific detachment', and incompetence becomes a 'lack of specialized

[34] MEADOR, Clifton. *The art and science of non-disease*, in: New England Journal of Medicine, 272, 1965, pp. 92–95. For the physician accustomed to dealing only with pathologic entities, terms such as 'non-disease entity' or 'non-disease' are foreign and difficult to comprehend. This paper presents a classification of non-disease and the important therapeutic principles based on this concept. Iatrogenic diseases probably arise as often from treatment of non-diseases as from the treatment of disease. BERGMAN, Abraham B., STAMM, Stanley J. *The morbidity of cardiac non-disease in school children*, in: The New England Journal of Medicine, Vol. 276, No. 18, May 4, 1967, gives one particular example from the 'limbo where people either perceive themselves or are perceived by others to have a non-existent disease. The ill effects accompanying some non-diseases are as extreme as those accompanying their counterpart diseases ... the amount of disability from cardiac non-disease in children is estimated to be greater than that due to actual heart disease.'

[35] Clinical iatrogenesis has a long history. PLINIUS SECUNDUS, *Naturalis Historia XXIX, 19*. 'To protect us against doctors there is no law against ignorance, no example of capital punishment. Doctors learn at our risk, they experiment and kill with sovereign impunity, in fact the doctor is the only one who may kill. They go further and make the patient responsible: they blame him who has succumbed.' In fact though, Roman law already contained some provisions against medically inflicted torts, 'damnum injuria datum per medicum'. Jurisprudence in Rome makes the doctor legally accountable not only for his ignorance and recklessness, but for bumbling. A doctor who has operated on a slave, but not properly followed up his convalescence, has to pay the price of the slave and the loss of income of the master during his protracted sickness. Citizens were not covered by these statutes, but could take action against the malpracticing doctor on their own.

[36] MONTESQUIEU. *De l'esprit des lois*. Livre XXIX, chap. XIV, b. Paris, Bibl. de la Pléiade, 1951. The Roman laws ordained that physicians should be punished for neglect or lack of skill (the Cornelian laws De Sicariis, Inst. iv, tit. 3, de lege Aquila 7). In those cases, if the physician was a person of any fortune or rank, he was only condemned to deportation, but if he was of low condition he was put to death. In our institutions it is otherwise. The Roman laws were not made under the same circumstances as ours: in Rome every ignorant pretender meddled with physics, but among us physicians are obliged to go through a regular course of study, and to take degrees, for which reason they are supposed to understand their profession.

equipment'. The depersonalization of diagnosis and therapy has turned malpractice from an ethical into a technical problem.

In 1971, between 12,000 and 15,000 malpractice suits were lodged in U.S. courts. However, doctors are vulnerable in court only to the imputation of having acted against the medical code, of having been guilty of the incompetent performance of prescribed treatment, or of dereliction out of greed or laziness. Most of the damage inflicted by the modern doctor does not fall into any of these categories. It occurs in the ordinary practice of well-trained men who have learned to bow to prevailing professional judgement and procedure, even though they know (or could and should know) what damage they do.

The U.S. Department of Health calculates that 7% of all patients suffer compensatable injuries while hospitalized, though few of them do anything about it. Moreover, the average frequency of reported accidents in hospitals was higher than in all industries but mines and high-rise construction. A national survey indicates that accidents were the major cause of death in U.S. children, and that these accidents occurred more often in hospitals than in any other kind of place.[37] One in 50 children admitted to a hospital suffered an accident which required specific treatment. University hospitals are relatively more pathogenic, or, in blunt language, more sickening. It has been established that one out of every five patients admitted to a typical research hospital acquires an iatrogenic disease, sometimes trivial, usually requiring special treatment, and in one case in thirty leading to death. Half of these episodes resulted from complications of drug therapy; amazingly, one in ten came from diagnostic procedures.[38] Despite good intentions and claims to public service, with a similar record of performance a military officer would be relieved of his command, and a restaurant or amusement centre would be closed by the police.

Defenceless Patients

The undesirable side-effects of approved, mistaken, callous or

[37] LOWREY, George H. *The problem of hospital accidents to children.* Reprinted from: Pediatrics, 32 (6): 1064–1068, December, 1963.

[38] MCLAMB, J. T. and HUNTLEY, R. R. *The hazards of hospitalization*, in: Southern Medical Journal, Vol. 60, May 1967, pp. 469–472.

contra-indicated technical contacts with the medical system represent only the first level of pathogenic medicine. This is 'clinical iatrogenesis'.[39] I include in this category not only those damages that doctors inflict with the intent of curing the patient or of exploiting him, but also those other torts which result from the doctor's attempt to protect himself against the patient's eventual suit of malpractice. 'Malpractice risks', to avoid litigation and prosecutions, may now do more damage than any other such iatrogenic stimulus.[40]

On a second level, medical practice sponsors sickness by reinforcing a morbid society that not only industrially preserves its defectives, but also exponentially breeds demand for the patient role. On the one hand defectives survive in increasing numbers and are fit only for life under institutional care, while on the other hand, medically certified symptoms exempt people from destructive wage-labour and excuse them from the struggle to reshape the society in which they live. Second level iatrogenesis finds its expression in various symptoms of social over-medicalization.[41] This second-level impact of medicine I will designate as *social iatrogenesis* and I shall discuss it in Part II.

On a third level, the so-called health professions have an even deeper, structurally health-denying effect insofar as they destroy the potential of people to deal with their human weakness, vulnerability and uniqueness in a personal and autonomous way.[42]

[39] AUDY, Ralph, *Man-made maladies and medicine*, in: California Medicine, November, 1970, 113–15, pp. 48–53, recognizes that iatrogenic diseases are only one type of man-made malady. According to their aetiology, they fall into several categories. Those resulting from diagnosis and treatment, those relating to social and psychological attitudes and situations, and those resulting from man-made programmes for the control and eradication of disease. Besides iatrogenic clinical entities, he recognizes other maladies that have a medical aetiology.

[40] Personal opinion expressed by Dr. Quentin YOUNG to the author.

[41] I use the term 'medicalization' in the sense coined by DUPUY. GREENBERG, Selig. *The quality of mercy. A report on the critical condition of hospital and medical care in America.* Foreword by Robert Ebert, N.Y., Atheneum, 1971, has used it in a different sense. For him society is 'overmedicated' because it spends too much on acquiring new medical knowledge and technique and too little to distribute it.

[42] HOKE, Bob. *Healths and healthing: beyond disease and dysfunctional environments.* Lecture at the annual meeting of the American Association for the Advancement of Science. Washington D.C., 29 December, 1972. 15 pp. summary in Ekistics, 220, March, 1974, pp. 169–172. Disease is an inevitable component of human life, so health as the absence of disease is an abstract and unattainable ideal ... It is unreasonable to think of health as a characteristic of man *per se*. Because man and environment constitute a system, health is a process of man-environment inter-

Structural iatrogenesis which I shall discuss in Part III is the ultimate backlash of hygienic progress and consists in the paralysis of healthy responses to suffering.[43] It strikes when people accept health management designed on the engineering model, when they conspire in an attempt to produce something called 'better health' which inevitably results in the heteronomous, managed maintenance of life on high levels of sub-lethal illness. This ultimate backlash of medical 'progress' must be clearly distinguished from both clinical and social iatrogenesis.

I hope to show that this three-tiered iatrogenesis has become medically irreversible. The unwanted physiological, social and psychological by-products of diagnostic and therapeutic progress have become resistant to medical remedies. New devices, approaches and organizational arrangements, which are conceived as remedies for clinical and social iatrogenesis, themselves tend to become pathogens contributing to the new epidemic. Technical and managerial measures taken to avoid damaging the patient by his treatment tend to engender a second order of iatrogenesis analogous to the escalating destruction generated by anti-pollution devices.[44]

---

action within a particular ecological context ... the assumption that good adjustment or adaptation to the environment is the only decisive factor in health makes some 'normal' events such as aging or adolescence into 'diseases' rather than phases or aspects of living which may have healthy ways of being lived ... There is a healthy way to live a disease.

[43] The sick in the grip of contemporary medicine is but a symbol of mankind in the grip of its technique. 'Das Schicksal das Kranken verkoerpert als Symbol das Schicksal der Menschheit im Stadium einer technischen Weltenwicklung.' JACOB, Wolfgang. *Der kranke Mensch in der technischen Welt.* IX. Internationaler Fortbildungakurs für praktische und wissenschaftliche Pharmazie der Bundesapothekerkammer in Meran. 1971. Werbe-und Vertriebsgesellschaft Deutscher Apotheker mbh. Frankfurt/Main.

[44] In the area of environmental degradation a conflict of two opposed approaches has already surfaced. On the one hand there are people who, like QUINN, James B. *Next big industry: environmental improvement*, in: Harvard Business Review, 49, Sept.–Oct., 1971, pp. 120–130, believe that environmental improvement is becoming a dynamic and profitable series of markets for industry that pay for themselves and in the end will represent an important addition to income and GNP. On the other hand people like DALY, Herman E. *Toward a steady state economy*, Freeman Co. 1973, distinguish two sections of the GNP, one represented by the value of directly desirable goods and services which reach the market, and another composed of the defensive expenditures needed to protect society against the values so created. For Daly only a radical decrease in industrial throughputs can save the environment. In medicine the bias is still overwhelmingly in favour of providing people with more,

I will designate this self-reinforcing loop of negative institutional feedback by its classical Greek equivalent and call it *medical nemesis*. The Greeks saw gods in the forces of nature. For them, nemesis represented divine vengeance visited upon mortals who infringe on those prerogatives the gods enviously guard for themselves. Nemesis is the inevitable punishment for inhuman attempts to be a hero rather than a human being. Like most abstract Greek nouns, Nemesis took the shape of a divinity. She represents nature's response to hubris: to the individual's presumption in seeking to acquire the attributes of a god. Our contemporary hygienic hubris has led to the new syndrome of medical nemesis.[45]

By using the Greek term I want to emphasize that the corresponding concept does not fit within the explanatory paradigm now offered by engineers, therapists and ideologues for the snowballing diseconomies, disutilities and counter-intuitive behaviour of large systems. By invoking myths and ancestral gods it should be clear that my framework for analysis of the current breakdown of medicine is foreign to any industrially determined logic and ethos.

Medical nemesis is resistant to medical care. It can be reversed only through a recovery of mutual self-care by the laity, and the legal, political and institutional recognition of this right to care. My final chapter proposes guidelines with which to stem medical nemesis and provides criteria by which the medical enterprise can be kept within healthy limits. It does not suggest any specific forms of health or sick-care and it does not advocate any new medical philosophy any more than it recommends remedies for diseases. I am not dealing with alternatives to any one medical technique, doctrine or organization, but with the alternative to this whole social enterprise and its allied bureaucracies and illusions.

---

although perhaps less risky, treatment. The need for a radical decrease in the total industrially produced service is not yet generally discussed in health, education or welfare.

[45] DAUMIER, Honoré (1810–1879). *Némésis médicale*. Drawing in: BLOCK, Werner, *Der Arzt und der Tod in Bildern aus sechs Jahrhunderten*, Stuttgart, Enbe Verlag, 1966.

PART II
SOCIAL IATROGENESIS

2 THE MEDICALIZATION OF LIFE

IN 1960 it would have been impossible to get a hearing for the claim that the ongoing medical endeavour itself was a bad thing. The National Health Service in Britain had just reached a high point in its development. It had been planned by Beveridge on the concepts of health prevailing in the 1930s. These assumed that there was a strictly 'limited quantity of morbidity', which if treated would result in a reduction in subsequent sickness rates. Thus Beveridge had expected that the annual cost of the health service would fall as effective therapy reduced morbidity.[46] It had not been expected that the definition of ill health would widen the scope of medical care and that the threshold of tolerance to disease would decline as fast as the competence for self-care or that new diseases would appear due to the same process that made medicine at least partially effective.

International co-operation had achieved its Pyrrhic victories over some tropical diseases. The role which economic and technological development would play in spreading and aggravating sleeping sickness, bilharzia and even malaria was not yet suspected.[47] The spectre of new types of rural and urban endemic hunger in 'developing' nations was still hidden. The risks of environmental degradation were still invisible to the public at large. In the U.S. people were getting ready to face the skyrocketing costs of care, the exorbitant privileges of doctors, and the inequitable access to their services.[48] Nationalization, or

[46] OFFICE OF HEALTH ECONOMICS. *Prospects in health*. OHE, 162 Regent Street, London W1R 6DD, 1971, 24 pp.

[47] For a survey of the literature on disease-consequences of developmental activities see HUGHES, Charles C., HUNTER, John M. *Disease and 'development' in Africa*, in: Social Science and Medicine, Vol. 3, No. 4, 1970, pp. 443-488.

[48] Neither had Edward Kennedy proposed that the federal government act as the insurance agent for the entire nation, covering all medical, dental and psychiatric costs without deductibles or upper limits, see KENNEDY, Edward M. *In critical condition: the crisis in America's health care*. N.Y., Simon and Shuster, 1972, nor had his opponents stated their case for an all-comprehensive Health Maintenance Organization. For a summary see ROY, William R. *The proposed health maintenance organization of 1972*. Washington, Science and Health Communications Group, Sourcebook Series, Vol. 2, 1972.

the replacement of privileged enterprise by regulated monopoly, still seemed the answer.[49] Everywhere the belief in unlimited progress was still unshaken, and progress in medicine meant the persistent effort to improve human health, abolish pain, eradicate sickness and extend the life span by using ever-new engineering interventions. Organ grafts, dialysis, cryogenics and genetic control still fired expectations rather than dread. The doctor was at the height of his role as a culture hero. The deprofessionalized use of modern medicine still had the status of a crank proposal.

By 1975 much has changed. People have learnt that health depends on the environment, on food and on working conditions, and that these, with economic development, easily turn into dangers to health, especially for the poor.[50] But people also still believe that health levels will improve with the amount spent on medical services, that more medical interventions would be better, and that doctors know best what these services should be.[51] People still trust the doctor with the key to the medicine cabinet and still value its contents, but increasingly they disagree on the manner in which doctors should be organized or controlled. Shall doctors be paid out of the individual's pocket, by insurance, or from taxes? Shall they practise as individuals or in groups? Shall they be accountable for health maintenance or for repairs? Shall the policy for health centres be set by specialists or by the community? In each case opposing parties still pursue the same goal of increasing the medicalization of health, albeit by different means. Too few, and the wrong kind of public controls over doctors, medicines, research,

[49] EHRENREICH, Barbara and John. *The American health empire: power, profits and politics*. A report from the Health Policy Advisory Center. N.Y., Random House, 1970.

[50] On the link between poverty and ill health in the U.S., see KOSA, John et al. eds. *Poverty and health: a sociological analysis*. A Commonwealth Fund Book, Cambridge, Mass., Harvard Univ. Press, 1969.

[51] STRICKLAND, Stephen P. *U.S. health care: what's wrong and what's right*. N.Y., Universe Books, 1972, 127 pp. A public opinion survey comes to the conclusion that 61% of the population and 68% of U.S. doctors are aware that basic changes are needed in the organization of U.S. medicine. Physicians rank the problems as: high cost of treatment, shortage of doctors, malpractice suits which hamper medical action, unnecessary hospitalization, limited insurance, rising expectation and lack of public education. The public blames shortage of doctors, costly and complicated insurance, unnecessary treatment, and doctors refusing house calls. The option of decreasing overall medicalization does not even enter the questions or the answers.

hospitals or insurance are blamed for current frustrations.[52]

In the meantime, total expectations increase faster than resources for care. Total suffering increases with more therapy. Total damages increase exponentially with the cost of care. More and more patients are told by their doctors that they have been damaged by previous medication and that the treatment now being given is conditioned by the consequences of their previous treatment, which sometimes had been given in a life-saving endeavour, and much more often for weight control, hypertension, flu or mosquito bite. A top official of the U.S. Department of Health could say that 80% of all funds channelled through his office provide no demonstrable benefits to health, and much of the rest is spent to offset iatrogenic damage. Economists might say that declining marginal utilities are dwarfed in comparison to the marginally rising disutilities produced by the medical endeavour. Soon the typical patient will come to understand that he is forced to pay more, not simply for less care, but for worse torts, for evil that he is the victim of, for damaging 'health production'—however well intentioned. For the time being, when people are hurt by the medical system, they are still believed to be exceptions. Rich people feel that they have had bad luck and poor people that they have been treated unjustly. But it is now only a matter of time before the majority of patients find out what epidemiological research discovers:[53] most of the time they would have been better off suffering without recourse to medicine. When this insight spreads, a sudden loss of

[52] To verify this summary on the overall trend of discussion, at least in the U.S.A., consult MARIEN, Michael, *World institute guide to alternative futures for health*, A bibliocritique of trends, forecasts, problems, proposals, draft, World Institute Council, N.Y., July, 1973, which is an annotated bibliography evaluating 612 books, articles and reports concerned with health policy in its broadest dimensions. The guide deals mainly with U.S. writings on U.S. subjects published or republished during the last 10 years. For France, consult MATHE, C. and G. *La santé est-elle au-dessus de nos moyens?* Paris, Plon, 1970.

[53] DINGLE, John H. *The ills of man*, in: Scientific American, 229, No. 3, Sept. 23, 1973, pp. 77–82. Opinions converge as to the ineffectiveness of medicine. The ills of man are differently perceived and defined in the perspective of the people still at large, the physician, the patient guided by the physician and by the keepers of vital statistics. From all four points of view the chief burden of man's ailments, numerically at least, consist of acute, benign, self-limiting illness. However, as longevity increases the chronic, degenerative diseases rapidly come to be the dominant cause not only of death but also of disability. On this too, the four distinct publics agree.

confidence might shake the present medical enterprise beyond repair.

During the last half dozen years, the attitudes of students towards their teachers have changed. It happened quite suddenly when students around 1968 admitted openly to each other what they had always known: that they learned from books, companions, cramming for examinations and a rare personal moment with a teacher, but not from the curricular system. Since then, many students have become consciously refractory to the teacher as an administrator of teaching procedures. The teacher became aware that he had lost respect, except on the rare occasions when he fell out of his role as a bureaucrat. It is not surprising, therefore, that at least in the U.S. and France, the drop-out rate among teachers has risen enormously.

When the crisis of confidence takes place in the medical system it will have deeper effects than the crisis in the school system. Students know that they will one day get out of school, the later the brighter their prospects. Patients, however, may come to feel that they might never get out of the hands of the doctors once having started on a patient career. Students who cynically accumulate certificates raise their chances on the job market, no matter how little they have learned. Patients will reasonably feel that they add to their original complaint not only new illnesses but also new certificates testifying to their job incompetence.

Today it is possible to foresee such a sudden crisis in health consciousness. The vague intuition of millions of victims of medical care requires clear concepts to gel into a powerful force. Without an intellectual framework, public recognition of iatrogenic medicine could easily lead to impotent anger which might be channelled by the profession to strengthen medical controls even further.[55] But if the experience of harm already done

[55] HOFFMAN, Allan., INGLIS, David Rittenhouse. *Radiation and infants*. A review of STERNGLASS, Ernest J. *Low level radiation*, in: Bulletin of the Atomic Scientists, December, 1972, pp. 45–52. The reviewers foresee the possibility of an imminent anti-scientific backlash from the general public when the kind of evidence provided by Sternglass becomes generally known. The public will come to feel that it has been lulled into a sense of security by unfounded optimism on the part of the spokesmen for scientific institutions with regard to the threat constituted by low level radiation. The reviewers argue for policy research to prevent such a backlash or to protect the scientific community from its consequences. I argue that a backlash against medicalization is equally imminent and that it will have characteristics that distinguish it

could be articulated in such clear, well-founded, and simply stated categories that would be useful in political discussion, it might endow entire populations with a new courage to recover their power for self-care.

The evidence needed for the indictment of our current medical system is not secret; it can be gleaned from prestigious medical journals and research reports.[56] It has not yet been put into political use, however, because it has not been properly gathered, clearly classified and presented in non-medical terms. The first task will be to suggest several categories of damage to health that are due to specific forms of medicalization. In each of these areas of over-medicalization, professional presumption and public credulity have reached health-denying levels.

Dependence on Care

One simple and obvious measure for the medicalization of life is the rising share of national budgets spent at the behest of doctors. The U.S. now spends 90 billion dollars a year for health care. This amount is equivalent to 17·4% of the GNP.[57] To assign a growing amount of national earnings to medicine, a country does not have to be rich. New Guinea, Nigeria and Jamaica are countries in which the medicalization of the budget has recently passed the 10% mark.

During the past 20 years, while the U.S. price index has risen by about 74%, the cost of medical care has escalated by 330%.[58]

---

clearly from a reaction against high-energy technology. The effects of a synergy of various iatrogenic pandemics will be directly observable by the general public. They will appear on a much shorter time-scale than the consequences of mutagenic radiation levels, and they will affect directly the quality of life of the observer rather than that of his offspring.

[56] BROOK, Robert, *Quality of care assessment: choosing a method for peer review* in: New England Journal of Medicine, Vol. 288, 1973, p. 1323ff. Depending on the method, from 1·4 to 63·2% of patients were judged to have received adequate care.

[57] MAXWELL, R. *Health care: the proving dilemma; needs versus resources in Western Europe, the US and the USSR*, Dekinsey & Co., N.Y., 1974.

[58] FELDSTEIN, Martin S. *The medical economy*, in: Scientific American, 229, No. 3, Sept. 1973, pp. 157–159, believes that the phenomenal rise in the cost of health services in the U.S. is due to the growing incidence of pre-payment for health services there. As a result of pre-payment, hospitals are moved towards increasingly expensive and new ways of doing things, rather than providing old products more efficiently and cheaply. Changing products rather than rising labour costs, bad

Most of the increase was paid out of an increased tax burden; while out-of-pocket payments for health services rose threefold, public expenditures for health rose exponentially. A good deal of this enriched not only doctors, but also bankers; the so-called administrative costs in the insurance business have risen to 70% of insurance payments to commercial carriers.

The rate of increase can be explained by rising costs of hospital care. The cost of keeping a patient for one day in a community hospital in the U.S. has risen 500% since 1950. The bill for patient care in major hospitals rose even faster: it tripled in eight years. Again, administrative expenses grew fastest, multiplying since 1964 by a factor of seven, laboratory costs by a factor of five.[59] Building a hospital bed now costs in excess of $85,000, of which two-thirds buys mechanical equipment written off or made redundant within ten years. There is no precedent for a similar expansion of a major sector of the civilian economy. It is ironic, therefore, that during this unique boom the U.S. witnessed another parallel event, also unprecedented in any industrial society: the life expectancy for adult American males declined, and is expected to decline even further.[60]

---

administration or lack of technological progress has caused this rise. One of the main reasons for this change in products is increased insurance coverage which encourages hospitals to provide more expensive products than the consumer actually wishes to purchase. His out-of-pocket costs appear increasingly modest, even though the service offered by the hospital is increasingly more costly. High cost hospital care is thus self-reinforcing. COHEN, Victor. *More hospitals to fill: abuses grow*, in: Technology Review, Oct.–Nov. 1973, pp. 14–16, deals with recent U.S. hospital building sprees and their effects. Since empty hospital beds in modern hospitals cost up to 66% of full beds, the filling of these beds becomes a major concern of a growing administration. This adds to the duplication of facilities and waste of complex equipment on people who cannot use it. Specialized personnel are spread thin. Medical standards are relaxed to keep the beds full, and unnecessary hospitalization leads to unnecessary surgery. See also LEE, M. L. *A conspicuous production theory of hospital behaviour*, in: Southern Economic Journal, July, 1971, pp. 48–58.

[59] KNOWLES, John J. *The hospital*, in: Scientific American, 229, No. 3, Sept. 1973, pp. 128–137.

[60] The trend is not limited to North America: LONGONE, P. *Mortalité et morbidité*, see note 1. Four factors characterize European mortality and morbidity today: mortality of adult males is stationary or increases; the relative life span of men as compared with women decreases, accidents increase as a cause of death, foetal and perinatal death claim 30% of conceptions. There is also lamentable lack of research on the subject. Accidents per 100,000 have not changed since 1900, but since other causes of death have declined, they have become more important.

In England the National Health Service ensured that the same kind of cost-inflation would be less plagued by conspicuous flim-flam. A stern commitment to equality prevented those astounding mis-allocations to prestigious gadgetry that have provided an easy starting point for public criticism in the U.S. Tight-fisted mis-allocations have made public criticism in the U.K. less colourful. While the life expectancy of adults in England has not yet declined, chronic diseases of middle-aged men have already shown an increase similar to that observed a decade earlier across the Atlantic. In the Soviet Union physicians and hospital days per capita have also more than tripled and costs have risen by 300% over the last 20 years.[61] All political systems generate the same dependence on physicians, even though capitalism imposes a much higher cost.

Only in China, at least at first sight, the trend seems to run in the opposite direction: primary care is given by non-professional health technicians assisted by health apprentices who leave their regular jobs in the factory when called to assist a member of their brigade.[62] In fact, however, the Chinese commitment to the ideology of technological progress is reflected already in the pro-fessional reaches of medical care. China possesses not only a para-medical system, but also medical personnel whose standards are known to be of the highest order by their counterparts around the world. Most investments during recent years have gone towards the further development of this extremely well qualified

[61] FIELD, Mark. *Soviet socialized medicine.* N.Y., Free Press, 1967.

[62] HORN, Joshua. *Away with all pests. An English surgeon in People's China, 1954–1969.* Monthly Review Press, 1969. SIDEL, Victor. *The barefoot doctors of the People's Republic of China*, in: The New England Journal of Medicine, June 15, 1972. SIDEL, Victor, SIDEL, Ruth. *The delivery of medical care in China.* The main feature of the Chinese system is an integrated network of neighbourhood stations that serve the functions of preventive medicine, primary medical care and referral to larger centres. in: Scientific American, Vol. 230, No. 4, April 1974, pp. 19–27. SELDON, Mark. *China: revolution and health.* Health/PAC Bulletin, No. 47, Dec. 1972. 20 pp. (Published by Health Policy Advisory Center, 17 Murray Street, New York, N.Y. 10007.) DJERASSI, Carl. *The Chinese achievement in fertility control.* One-third of the women of child-bearing age may be practising birth control, in: Bulletin of the Atomic Scientists, June, 1974, pp. 17–24. FOGARTY INTERNATIONAL CENTER, *A bibliography of Chinese sources on medicine and public health in the People's Republic of China: 1960–1970.* DHEW Publication No. (NIH) 73–439. LIN, Paul T. K. *Medicine in China*, in: The Center Magazine, May/June, 1974. LIANG, et al. *Chinese health care. Determinants of the system*, in: American Journal of Public Health, Vol. 63, No. 2, p. 102 ff. February 1973.

and very orthodox medical profession; 'barefoot medicine' is increasingly losing its makeshift, semi-independent character and is being integrated into a unitary health care system. After a short honeymoon with a radical deprofessionalization of health care, the system of referral from the neighbourhood through several levels of increasingly more complex hospitals has grown at a remarkable speed. I believe that this development of a technical-professional side of medical care in China would have to be consciously limited in the very near future if it were to remain a balancing complement rather than an obstacle to high-level self-care.

The proportion of national wealth which is channelled to doctors and expended under their control varies from one nation to another, and falls between one-tenth and one-twentieth of all available funds. This means that the average expenditure per capita varies by a factor of up to 1,000: from about $320 in the U.S. through $9·60 in Jamaica to $0·40 in Nigeria.[63] Most of this money is spent everywhere on the same kinds of things. But the poorer the country, the higher the unit price tends to be. Modern hospital beds, incubators, laboratory equipment or respirators cost even more in Africa than in Germany or France where they are made; they break down more easily in the tropics, are difficult to service, and are more often out of use. The same is true for the investment in the training of doctors who use such highly capitalized equipment. The education of a cardiologist represents a comparable capital investment whether he comes from a socialist school system or is the cousin of an industrialist in Brazil sent on a government scholarship to study in Germany. The poorer the country, the greater the concentration of rising medical expenditures. Beyond a certain point, which may vary from country to country, intensive treatment of the patient requires the concentration of large sums of public funds to provide a very few with the doubtful privileges doctors confer. This concentration of public resources is obviously unjust when the ability to pay for a small fraction of the total cost of treatment is a condition for getting the remainder underwritten by tax funds. It is clearly a form of exploitation when about 80% of the real costs of private

[63] BRYANT, John H. *Health and the developing world.* Ithaca, London, Cornell Univ. Press, 1971.

clinics in poor Latin American countries are paid for by taxes collected for the education of doctors, the operation of ambulances, and the price-support of medical equipment. In socialist countries, the public assigns to doctors alone the power to decide who 'needs' this kind of treatment, and to reserve lavish public support to those on whom they experiment or practice. The recognition of the doctor's ability to identify needs only broadens the base from which doctors can sell their services.[64]

This professionally consecrated favouritism, however, does not constitute the most important aspect of the mis-allocation of funds. The concentration of resources on a cancer hospital in São Paolo might deprive dozens of villages in the Mato Grosso of any chance for a small clinic, but it does not undermine the ability of people to care for themselves. Public support for a nationwide addiction to therapeutic relationships is pathogenic on a much deeper level, but this is usually not recognized. More health damages are caused by the belief of people that they cannot cope with illness without modern medicines than by doctors who foist their ministrations on patients.

Handbooks that deal with iatrogenesis concentrate overwhelmingly on the clinical variety. They recognize the doctor as a pathogen alongside resistant strains of bacteria, hospital corridors, poisonous pesticides, and badly engineered cars. It has not yet been recognized that the proliferation of medical institutions, no matter how safe and well engineered, unleashes a social pathogenic process. Over-medicalization changes adaptive ability into passive medical consumer discipline.

An analogy with the transportation system might clarify the dangers of over-medicalization so clearly reflected in the budget. No doubt cars are dangerous. They kill more than one-quarter of those in the U.S. who die between childhood and the age of 60. If drivers were better educated, laws better enforced, vehicles better constructed and roads better planned, fewer people would die in cars. The same could be said about doctors: they are dangerous. If doctors were differently organized, if patients were better educated by them, for them and with them, if the

[64] FUCHS, Victor. *The contribution of health services to the American economy*, in: Milbank Memorial Fund Quarterly. Vol. XLIV, 4, Part II, October 1966, pp. 65–103.

hospital system were better planned, the accidents which now result from contact between people and the medical system could be reduced.

But the reason why high speed transportation now produces accidents lies deeper than the kind of cars people drive, and even deeper than the decision to depend for locomotion mainly on cars, rather than on buses or trains. It is not the choice of the vehicle but the decision to organize modern society around high-speed transportation which turns locomotion from a healthy activity into a health-denying form of consumption. No matter how well constructed the vehicle, or how well programmed the landing, at some point of acceleration the rhythm of the machine will destroy the rhythm of life. At a given point of acceleration, things and the people strapped to them begin to move in an engineered time-space continuum which is biologically anti-thetical to that for which the human animal has evolved. The more hurried a crowded world becomes, the higher must be the incidence of trauma which results from unhealthy encounters, violent separation, and enervating restraint. Vehicles become unhealthy when they compel people to speed. It is not their specific construction or the choice of a private car over a public bus that makes transportation unhealthy, but their speed itself and the intensity of their use.

This health-denying aspect of the speedup in traffic is generally not taken into account when the health dangers of traffic are discussed. In a bibliography of Traffic Medicine[65] listing 6,000 items, I did not find one paper dealing with the impact of acceleration on health. The same applies to bibliographies on iatrogenic diseases. More than one thousand items are listed each year under this title in the standard Index Medicus. People with a penchant for the grotesque might enjoy reading the gory details, but they will not find any mention of the health-denying effect of a growing dependence on medical care.

The proliferation of medical agents is health-denying not only or primarily because of the specific functional or organic lesions produced by doctors, but because they produce dependence. And this dependence on professional intervention tends to impoverish

[65] HOFFMAN, Herman. *Ausgewählte internationale Bibliographie 1952–1963 zur Verkehrsmedizin*. München, Lehman 1967.

the non-medical health-supporting and healing aspects of the social and physical environments, and tends to decrease the organic and psychological coping ability of ordinary people. Modern apartments are increasingly unfit for the sick, and family members are often frightened by the idea that they might be asked to care for their own sick.[66]

Dependence on Drugs

Doctors are not needed to sponsor addiction to medicine. Poor countries that cannot afford widespread dependence on professionals nevertheless produce sickness from the compulsive use of prescription drugs. Twenty years ago half as many drug varieties were marketed in Mexican pharmacies as in the U.S. In 1962 the U.S. law that drugs had to be proven effective and not only safe brought the proliferation of medicines under some kind of control. In Mexico there are now four times as many drugs on sale as in the U.S.: about 80,000 distinct items are marketed and their packaging has become nondescript. Ten years ago, each drug came packaged with a descriptive leaflet written in the language of doctors and useless for the rural majority who had to rely on their instincts. But drugs were scarce and people poor; most of them still relied on their herbalist. Today drugs are more plentiful, more effective, and more dangerous, and people who earn a little more have been taught to feel ashamed of their trust in Aztec herbalists and dietary rules. The leaflet has disappeared and has been replaced by an identical statement on the containers of insulin, vitamins, and sleep and birth control pills: 'to be used only under medical supervision'. Such counsel, of course, is merely a pious gesture because there are not enough doctors in Mexico to prescribe antibiotics for every case of salmonellosis, nor pharmacies which insist on prescriptions. With the advent of

[66] The medicalization of care has a profound impact on the structure of contemporary man-made space. The empire of the health professions is cemented into modern society. The forthcoming book by Roslyn LINDHEIM (Calder and Boyars, 1975) will demonstrate this. For the moment consult: LINDHEIM, Roslyn. *New environment for births*. Manuscript at CIDOC, 1971. *Humanization of medical care: an architect's view*. Third draft. April 1, 1974. *Environments for the elderly. Future-oriented design for living?* Febr. 20, 1974, mimeo.

effective chemical agents, the function of the physician in developing countries becomes increasingly trivial; most of the time he is reduced to prescribing without previous clinical tests.[67] He comes to feel useless even in his trivial function because he knows that more and more people will use the same kind of drug not only without tests but also without his approval. As drugs are being made increasingly into tools legally and technically reserved to the doctor, people are more prone to damage themselves medically with these drugs, with or without a prescription. The medicalization of a drug renders it in fact more dangerous. Chloromycetin is a good example: for a decade it was prescribed against typhoid against which it is effective, and also for many other conditions, against which it is not and, as a result, aplastic anaemia became quite common. At the same time, the absence of a clear warning about the dangers of the drug led people to use it on their own even when other treatment would have been quite as effective. Thus doctors and patients collaborated in the breeding of drug-resistant strains of typhoid bacilli now spreading from Mexico to the rest of the world.[68]

Dr. Salvador Allende, the late President of Chile who was also a physician, has so far been the only Latin American statesman who has tried to stem progressive drug abuse.[69] He proposed forbidding the importation of new drugs into Chile unless they had first been tested on the North American public for at least seven years without being withdrawn by the U.S. Food and Drug Administration. He also proposed a reduction of the national pharmacopeia to a few dozen items, more or less the same ones carried by each Chinese 'barefoot doctor'. By far the majority of Chilean doctors resisted the call of their president; many of the minority who tried to translate his ideas into practical pro-

[67] ALDAMA, Arturo. *Establecimiento de un laboratorio farmacéutico nacional*, in: Higiene, Organo Oficial de la Sociedad de Higiene. Vol. XI, No. 1, January/February, 1959.
[68] SCHREIER, Herbert and BERGER, Lawrence, *On medical imperialism*. A letter in: LANCET, 1974, v I. p. 1161. 'Under pressure from the U.S. Food and Drug Administration, Parke Davis inserted strict warnings of hazards and cautionary statements about indications for the use of the drug in the U.S.A. The warnings did not extend to the same drug sold abroad.'
[69] WAITZKIN, Howard and MODELL, Hilary, *Medicine, socialism and totalitarianism: Lesson from Chile*. New England Journal of Medicine, 291: 171–177, 1974.

grammes were murdered within one week after the take-over by the junta on September 11, 1973.[70]

The over-consumption of *medical drugs* is not restricted to areas where doctors are scarce. In the U.S., central nervous system agents are the fastest growing sector in the pharmaceutical market, making up 31% of total sales.[71] Dependence on prescribed tranquillizers has risen by 290% since 1962, a period during which the per capita consumption of liquor rose by only 23% and the estimated consumption of illegal opiates by about 50%.[72] Medicalized addiction outgrew all self-chosen forms.

Over-prescription in capitalist economies[73] is a pet argument for people who want to right the wrongs of medicine by public controls of the drug industry. According to these critics, the indiscriminate medication in the U.S. or in France can best be explained by the pressure which pharmaceutical firms

[70] JONSEN, Albert, et al. *Doctors in Politics: a lesson from Chile*, in: New England Journal of Medicine, August 29, 1974, pp. 471–472. 'Physicians identified and denounced colleagues whom they considered politically unacceptable. Lists were prepared throughout the country and may have resulted in the death of some 15 doctors. Almost 300 physicians were arrested and held for long periods without charges. Many of these were physically abused. The National Health Service still has lists containing the names of 2,100 health workers, of whom 130 are physicians. Their professional future is in serious doubt. Probably 250 physicians have fled Chile since the coup because their political views are unacceptable.'

[71] GODDARD, James L. *The medical business*, in: Scientific American, 229, No. 3, Sept., 1973, pp. 161–166. Goddard provides good graphs and charts showing U.S. sales of non-prescription and prescription drugs by category 1962–71; breakdown of sales dollar estimated in 1968 for 17 leading pharmaceutical houses, introduction of new drugs, combinations and dosage forms 1958–72. He also identifies 8 classes of prescription drugs. Within the category of 'nervous system drugs' alone there are more than one billion per year. Three other categories each had about half a billion, and four categories had less than 350 million. Prescriptions per capita increased by 150% in 10 years. LEVINSON, Charles. *Valium zum Beispiel. Die multinationalen Konzerne der pharmazeutischen Industrie*. Rowohlt Taschenbuch, 1974. Levinson has gathered information on pricing and marketing policies in the drug industry. YURICK, Sol. *The political economy of junk*, in: Monthly Review, Dec., 1970, pp. 22–37. Yurick first suggested that addictive drugs have generated a huge infra-economy in which the government is spending many times as much as the addicts.

[72] NATIONAL COMMISSION ON MARIJUANA AND DRUG ABUSE. *Marijuana: a signal of misunderstanding*. First report of the Commission. Washington, U.S. General Printing Office, 1972, 2 vols. The report has never been made publicly available. It seems to conclude that rising addiction to alcohol is the most serious problem of addiction.

[73] BALTER, Mitchell, et al. *Cross-national study of the extent of anti-anxiety/sedative drug use*, in: New England Journal of Medicine, April 4, 1974, pp. 769–774, provides evidence of high uniformity in use in U.S. and nine European countries.

exercise on overworked clinicians. They point out that U.S. physicians receive their most intensive in-service training from agents of the chemical industry. On each of the 350,000 practising physicians, the industry spent in 1972 $4,500 on advertising and promotion.[74] Surprisingly, however, the per capita use of medically prescribed tranquillizers correlates with per capita income all over the world, even in socialist countries, where the recurrent education of doctors is not accounted for as 'publicity' by private industry. Increasingly, the doctor is working with two groups of drug addicts: in one he prescribes addictive drugs, and in the other he is responsible for the care of people who are suffering from the consequences of having drugged themselves.[75] The richer the community, the larger the percentage of his patients who belong simultaneously to both.[76]

Medicalization of the Life Span

The medicalization of life appears as the encroachment of health-care on the budget, the dependence on professional care, and as the addiction to medical drugs; it also takes form in iatrogenic labelling of the ages of man. This labelling becomes part of a culture when laymen accept it as a trivial verity that people require routine medical ministrations for the simple fact that they are unborn, newborn, infants, in their climacteric, or old. When this happens, life turns from a succession of different stages of health into a series of periods each requiring different therapies. Each age then demands its own health-producing environment: from the crib to the workplace, to the retirement home and the terminal ward. In each place people are made to follow a special medical routine. This specialization degrades the quality of the home, the school, the street and the market place. The doctor's

[74] PEKKANEN, John. *The American connection*, Follett Publishing Co. Chicago, 1973, gives information on advertising costs in American drug firms.

[75] FREEDMAN, Alfred M. *Drugs and society: an ecological approach*, in: Comprehensive Psychiatry, Vol. 13, No. 5, Sept.–Oct., 1972, pp. 411–420.

[76] FORD FOUNDATION. *Dealing with drug abuse: a report to the Ford Foundation*. N.Y., Praeger, 1972. This report concludes that potentially addictive drugs will inevitably be available in growing varieties. The attempt to suppress these substances or to repress their unauthorized use cannot but increase drug-induced violence, while their prescription inevitably will increase the possibilities for their abuse.

grasp over life starts with the monthly pre-natal check-up when he decides if and how the foetus shall be born; it ends with his decision to abandon further resuscitation. The environment comes to be seen as a mechanical womb and the health professional as the bureaucrat who assigns to each his proper corner.

The chief burden of man's ailments, numerically at least, consists of illness which is acute and benign—either self-limiting or limited by a few dozen routine interventions. Disease itself is largely self-limiting.[77] With regard to a wide range of conditions, those who are treated least probably make the best progress. More often than not, the best a conscientious physician can do is to console his patient that he can live with his impairment, perhaps reassure him about an eventual recovery, do what his grandmother could have done for him, and otherwise defer to nature. The fact that modern medicine has become very effective for specific symptoms does not mean that it has become more beneficial for the health of the patient.

This is true for conditions which have long been recognized as sickness, such as flu, rheumatism and many tropical diseases. It is even more true when the condition has only recently been put under medical control. Old age, for example, is not a disease in this sense, but recently it has been medicalized. The average life-span has increased. Many more children survive, no matter how sickly and needy of special institutional care. The life expectancy of young adults has increased, notwithstanding the high rate of mortal accidents, because they survive pneumonias and other infections. But the maximum life-span has not changed at all. Old people become increasingly prone to be ill. No matter how much medicine they take, no matter what care is given to them, life expectancy by the age of 65 has remained practically unchanged over the last century. Medicine cannot do much for illness associated with aging, and even less about the process of aging itself. It cannot cure cardiovascular diseases, most cancers, arthritis, advanced cirrhosis, or the common cold.[78] It is true that some of the pain which the aged suffer can sometimes be

---

[77] GINZBERG, Eli. *Men, money and medicine*. N.Y., Columbia University Press, 1969.
[78] EXTON-SMITH, A. N. *Terminal illness in the aged*, in: Lancet, 2, 1961, p. 305. In the geriatric unit studied, 82% of those with fatal illness died within three months of admission.

45

lessened. Unfortunately though, most treatment of the old requiring professional intervention not only tends to heighten their pain, but, if successful, also protracts it.[79] The support of one vital system often brings into prominence a more awkward or painful disorder.

10% of the U.S. population is over 65. 28% of health care is spent on this minority. What is more, this minority is outgrowing the remainder of the population at an annual rate of 3%, while the per capita cost of their care is rising at a rate of 5% to 7% faster than overall per capita care.[80] Parallel with and due to this medicalization of age is a decline in the opportunities for independent aging. The reinterpretation of old age as a geriatric 'problem' has cast the elderly in the role of a minority who must feel painfully deprived of necessities at any level of relative privilege.[81] What medicalization has done to old age it does with equal effectiveness to people who are pregnant, are addicted to heroin or methadone, go through the menopause, or are alco-

---

[79] Nursing homes often lessen pain by shortening life: JUTMAN, David. *The hunger of old men*, in: Transaction. Nov. 12, 1971, pp. 55–66. The mortality rate during the first year of living in a home for the aged is significantly higher than the mortality rate of those staying on in their usual surroundings: PATTON, R. G.; GARDNER, L. I. *Growth failure in maternal deprivation*. Springfield, Ill., Charles C. Thomas, 1963. Some old people seem to choose the old-age home to shorten their lives: MARKSON, Elizabeth, *A hiding place to die*, in: Transaction, Nov. 12, 1972, pp. 48–54. Separation from the family and recovery in an institution is a contributing factor to the appearance of serious diseases, including asthma, cancer, congestive heart failure, diabetes mellitus, disseminated lupus eythematosus, functional uterine bleeding, Raynaud's disease, rheumatoid arthritis, thyrotoxicosis, tuberculosis and ulcerative colitis. For bibliography on each, see BAKAN, David. *Disease, pain and sacrifice. Toward a psychology of suffering*. Boston, Beacon Press, 1971. Often the disease triggered by or related to separation has an above average rate of mortality.

[80] FORBES, W. H. *Longevity and medical costs*, in: New England Journal of Medicine, July 13, 1967. MORISON, Robert S. *Dying*, in: Scientific American, 229, No. 3, Sept., 1973.

[81] BEAUVOIR, Simone de. *La vieillesse*. Gallimard, 1970. For the sociology of aging and the relevant bibliography see BIRREN, James E., TALMON, Yonina, CHEIT, Earl F. *Aging. I. Psychological aspects. II. Social aspects. III. Economic aspects*, in: International Encyclopedia of Social Sciences, 1968, Vol. 1, pp. 176–202. ROEHLAU, Volkmar, ed. *Wege zur Erforschung des Alterns*, Vol. 189 in Wege der Forschung. Wissenschaftliche Büchergesellschaft, 1973. A representative selection of 30 recent German contributions to geriatrics. AMERY, Jean. *Über das Altern. Revolte und Resignation*. Stuttgart, Ernst Klett Verlag, 1968. An exceptionally sensitive phenomenology of aging. GUILLEMARD, Anne-Marie. *La retraite une mort sociale. Sociologie des conduites en situation de retraite*. Paris, Mouton, 1972. A socio-economic study which demonstrates that class-discrimination is accentuated in retirement.

holics. They constitute a special clientele and often graduate from one specialist to the next. The public acceptance of iatrogenic labelling multiplies patients faster than either doctors or drugs can medicalize them.

In poor countries the medicalization of the ages of man is often euphemistically called the 'process of modernization'.[82] In 1960, 96% of Chilean mothers breast-fed their babies beyond the first year. By 1970 only 6% did so, and only 20% nursed their babies as long as two full months. Chilean women went through a period of intense political indoctrination given by both right-wing Christian Socialists and left-wing parties. As a result of this modernization, 84% of potential human breast milk remains unproduced. The milk of about 32,000 Chilean cows would be required to compensate for that loss, which was the result of a new concern for the mother's health and the child's access to a complete formula approved by the doctor.[83] As the bottle became a status symbol, new medical attention became necessary, because new illnesses appeared among children who had been denied the breast, and mothers lacked the know-how to deal with children who were not behaving as breast-fed children do.[84]

Medicalization of Prevention

As curative treatment has focused increasingly on conditions in which it is ineffective, expensive and painful, the prevention of sickness by the intervention of body maintenance men has become a fad. After sick care, health care has become a commodity, something one gets rather than something one does. The higher the salary the company pays, or the higher the rank of an aparatchnik, the more will be spent to keep such a valuable cog well oiled. The consumption of health care is the new status

---

[82] BERG, Alan. *The nutrition factor: its role in national development*. Washington, Brookings Institution, 1973. A child nursed through the first two years of its life receives the nutritional equivalent of 461 quarts of cow's milk, which costs the equivalent of the average yearly income of an Indian.

[83] From a study in the CIDOC file. Also: WADE, Nicolas, Science 1974.

[84] The pattern of world-wide modern malnutrition is reflected in the two forms which infant malnutrition takes: while the switch from the breast to the bottle introduces Chilean babies to a life of endemic under-nourishment, the same switch initiates British babies to a life of sickening over-alimentation see: OATES, R. K. *Infant feeding practices*, in: British Medical Journal, 1973, 2, pp. 762–764.

symbol for the middle classes. People today keep up with the Joneses by having just as many 'check-ups': the English word 'check-up' is now part of the everyday vocabulary in French, Serbian, Spanish, Malay and Hungarian. The extension of professional control over the care of healthy people is another expression of the medicalization of life. People have become patients without being sick.[85] The medicalization of prevention is a fourth major symptom of social iatrogenesis.

Over the last decade, a number of doctors heralded a revolution in medicine through new methods of professional health maintenance for the masses. They got support not only from aging statesmen, but also from the leaders with a large popular following who were envious of a privilege so far reserved to the rich. Monthly pre-natal visits became fashionable, along with clinics for infants who were well, school[86] and camp check-ups and pre-paid medical schemes to provide early diagnosis as well as preventative therapies.[87]

The development of automated multiphasic health testing is seen by some as a panacea. This assembly-line procedure of complex chemical and medical tests can be performed by non-professional technicians at a surprisingly low cost. It purports to offer for uncounted millions a more sophisticated detection of hidden therapeutic needs than was available in the sixties even for a few very 'valuable' people in Houston or Moscow. The lack of controlled studies at the outset of this testing has allowed the salesmen of prevention to foster unsubstantiated expectations. Controlled comparative studies of population groups benefiting from maintenance service and early diagnosis have only recently become available. So far, a review of two dozen studies shows that

[85] DUPUY, Jean-Pierre. *Relations entre dépenses de santé, mortalité.* Paris, CEREBE., April 1973. 'The concept of morbidity has simply been extended and is applied to situations which have nothing to do with morbidity in the strict sense but merely with the probability that morbidity may appear within a given time . . . the patient who consults his doctor about a condition which appears to be abnormal is "ill" to the same extent as the patient who consults his doctor about a symptom which is morbid in the strict sense of the word.' p. 31.

[86] YANKAUER, Alfred., LAWRENCE, Ruth A. *A study of periodic school medical examinations,* in: American Journal of Public Health, 45, Jan., 1955, pp. 71–78. Does not indicate significant value.

[87] WYLIE, C. M. *Participation in a multiple screening clinic with five year follow-up,* in: Public Health Reports, 76, July, 1961. pp. 596–602. Indicates disappointing results.

these diagnostic procedures—even when followed by high-level medical therapy—have no impact on life expectancy.

The truth is that early diagnosis transforms people who feel healthy into anxious patients.[88] To begin with, there are serious risks associated with some diagnostic procedures. Cardiac catheterization, a test to determine if a patient suffers from cardiomyopathy, admittedly not done routinely, kills one in fifty people on whom it is performed.[89] It is done at a cost of $350 per patient, even though no evidence has been shown so far that a differential diagnosis based on its results extends either the life expectancy or the comfort of the patient. Most tests are less murderous and many do provide guidance for the choice of therapy, but when associated with others each has a greater power to harm than any one by itself. Even if people survive a positive laboratory diagnosis unharmed, they have incurred a very high risk of being submitted to therapy that is odious, painful, crippling and expensive. Ironically, the serious asymptomatic disorders which this kind of screening alone can discover are frequently incurable illnesses in which early treatment aggravates the patient's physical condition.

Routine performance of early diagnostic tests on large populations guarantees the medical scientist a broad base from which to select the cases that best fit existing treatment facilities or are most effective in the attainment of research goals, whether or not the therapies cure, rehabilitate or soothe. In the process, people are strengthened in their belief that they are machines whose durability depends on visits to the maintenance shop, and are obliged to pay for the market research and the sales activities of the medical establishment.

The medicalization of prevention fosters the confusion of prevention with insurance. Only when a thing has no value other than its dollar equivalent can one apply the definition for

[88] SIEGEL, G. S. *The uselessness of periodic examination*, in: Archives of Environmental Health, 13, Sept. 1966, pp. 292–295. CLOTE, Paul D. *Automated multiphasic health testing*. An evaluation. Independent study with John McKnight, Northwestern University, 1973. Reproduced in CIDOC *Antologia A8*, Cuernavaca, 1974.

[89] Such a procedure is as informative as recording a patient's blood pressure once in a lifetime, or examining his urine once every 20 years. This practice is ridiculous, absurd and unnecessary . . . and of absolutely no value in diagnosis or treatment. PAPPWORTH, Maurice. *Dangerous head that may rule the heart*, in: Perspective, p. 67–70.

'insurance' given in an American dictionary, according to which 'we insure to protect ourselves against loss'. In fact, no insurance company can protect us against the loss of car, house, health or life. The broker cannot prevent any of these from being destroyed. All he can offer is the payment of a certain sum if we suffer a loss. Driving is no safer because the premium is paid up. Even if there were substance to the myth that costly medical treatment can restore health or prolong life, insurance cannot protect against sickness or death. Yet, as a study in Chicago shows, the more years of schooling people have absorbed, the more intensely they defend the thesis that their health will be better if they are insured.[90]

Effective health care depends on self-care: this fact is currently heralded as if it were a discovery. But equally, the early discovery of those few degenerative diseases in which the patient could find relief as a result of early medical intervention depends in most cases on the patient's own recognition of a probable symptom of serious illness. Scheduled yearly medical check-ups for the detection of most early cancers come too late because they are spaced too far apart.[91] People who are told by their doctors that their heart is in good shape and are thus encouraged to continue an unhealthy rhythm of living are probably more numerous than people who are helped by their doctor's advice when they are in trouble. The medicalization of early diagnosis not only hampers and discourages preventative health-care but it also trains the patient-to-be to function in the meantime as an acolyte to his doctor.[92] He learns to depend on the physician in sickness and in health. He turns into a life-long patient.

[90] Personal communication from John MCKNIGHT on an inquiry at Northwestern University in Evanston, Illinois.

[91] See footnote 88, CLOTE, Paul D.

[92] COOPER, Joseph, *A non-physician looks at medical utopia*, in: Journal of American Medical Association, Aug. 29, 1966, pp. 105–107, formulates in journalistic style the consequences of the ultimate medical programme in a systems society, where the total service of health could become the main activity of an inner-directed nation. By equating statistical man with biologically unique men, an insatiable demand for finite resources is created. The individual is subordinated to the greater needs of the whole. Preventative procedures become compulsory, and the right of the patient to consent to his own treatment is increasingly withdrawn in the face of the argument that society cannot afford the burden of more expensive curative procedures.

Medicalization of Expectations

Like any other growth industry, the health system directs its products where the demand seems unlimited: into defence against death. The medicalization of major rituals constitutes a fifth important symptom of social iatrogenesis. An increasing percentage of newly acquired tax funds is allocated towards life-extension technology for terminal patients.[93] 'Consultants' sanctimoniously select one in every five of those Englishmen who are afflicted with kidney failure and condition him to desire the scarce privilege of dying in protracted torture on dialysis. Much time and effort during the treatment is used in the prevention of suicide during the first and sometimes the second year that the artificial kidney may add to the lives of patients.[94]

Again intensive cardiac care units are other gadgets which have high visibility and no proven advantage for the care of the sick. They require three times the equipment and five times the staff needed for normal patient care. 12% of all graduate hospital nurses in the U.S. now work in these units. The equipment has become an international symbol for peaceful progress ever since Nixon and Brezhnev agreed to co-operate in the conquest of space, cancer and heart disease. The gaudy care is financed, like the liturgies of old, by taxes, gifts and sacrifices.[95] Large-scale randomized samples have been used for comparison of the mortality and recovery rates of patients served by these units with those of patients given home treatment. So far they have demonstrated no advantage. The patients who have suffered

[93] For bibliography see note 233.

[94] CALLAND, G. H. *Iatrogenic problems in end stage renal failure*, in: New England Journal of Medicine, 287–334, 1972. This is the autobiographical account of a medical doctor in such terminal treatment.

[95] The deep-rooted reasons for the existence of such torture in our society might have to be sought in a symbolic rather than medical or merely economic need. HENTIG, Hans von. *Vom Ursprung der Henkersmahlzeit*, Tübingen, Mohr, 1958, is an encyclopaedic study of the condemned man's breakfast in a great variety of cultures. A deep-felt need exists to lavish favours on persons who are to die under public control. It usually takes the form of a lavish meal. In our century it has been reduced frequently to a last cigarette. The modern soldier, who is trained to kill rather than to fight, is the first executioner who does not meet his victim as a person. Terminal treatment has been depersonalized in war as in medicine. Ritual execution of a death sentence might not only take the form of judicial murder but also of the discontinuation of terminal care. The sumptuous treatment of the comatose then takes the place of the condemned man's breakfast.

51

cardiac infarcts themselves tend to express a preference for home care. They are frightened by the hospital, and in a crisis would rather be close to people they know. Careful statistical findings have confirmed their intuition.[96] Some patients in these units understandably suffer acute psychoses.

Public fascination with 'medical breakthroughs', high-technology care, and death under medical control is a fifth symptom of the intense medicalization of our culture. It can best be understood as a deep-seated need for miracle cures. High-technology medicine is the most solemn element in a ritual celebrating and reinforcing the myth that doctors struggle heroically against death.[97] The willingness of the public to finance these activities corresponds to a need for the non-technological functions of medicine.[98]

Technical intervention in the physical and biochemical make-up of the patient or his environment is not, however, and never has been, the sole function of medical institutions. The application of remedies, effective or not, is by no means the only way of mediating between man and his disease. Magic, or healing through the impact of ceremonial, is certainly one among several important functions medicine has served. Magic works because the intent of patient and magician coincide.[99]

[96] MATHER, H. G., PEARSON, N. G., READ, K. L. G. et al. *Acute myocardial infarction: home and hospital treatment*, in: British Medical Journal, 3, 1971, pp. 334–338. LOCKWOOD, Howard J. et al. *Effects of intensive care on the mortality rate of patients with myocardial infarctions*, in: Public Health Reports, 78, Aug., 1963. pp. 655–661.

[97] Fear of an un-medicalized death is becoming quite common. In most Western countries hospital deaths, which made up one-third of total deaths after World War I, now make up more than two-thirds. People tend to think that they have a high probability of spending an extended period in the hospital before death, and that this will reduce their suffering. Evidence does not support this belief. HINTON, John. *Dying*. Penguin Books, 1974. In teaching hospitals studied by the author, 10% of those admitted with a condition which would prove fatal died on their first day in the hospital. 30% died within a week, 75% within a month and nearly all (97%) deaths took place within three months. 40% of all fatalities except cancer occurred within 7 days of the patient entering the hospital. In homes for the dying 56% die within the first week of admission.

[98] POWLES, John. See note 43. A large, increasing proportion of contemporary disease burden is man-made; engineering intervention in sick persons is not making much progress as a strategy. Insistence on it can be explained only if it serves non-technical purposes. Diminishing returns within medicine is a specific instance of a wider crisis in industrial man's relationship to his environment.

[99] GOODE, William J. *Religion and magic*, in: Religion among the primitives. Free Press, 1951, pp. 50–54. Magic is distinct from religion because it is more a concrete,

Religious medicine is something else again. Great religions have always provided the social reinforcement of resignation to misfortune by offering a rationale and a style for dignified suffering. Suffering can be explained, for instance, as Karma accumulated through a past incarnation, or can be made valuable by interpreting it as a close association with the Saviour on the Cross. A third important non-technical function of medical procedures is the training of the community for dealing with the sick. By assigning an active role to community members, the suffering of the diseased can be lessened. Cultures where compassion for the unfortunate, hospitality for the cripple, and tolerance for the madman have been well developed, can, to a large extent, integrate those who are ill into everyday life.

Among these many functions of medicine, one has recently overshadowed all others. It is the attempt to manage all diseases by means of engineering interventions. Paradoxically, the more attention was focused on the technical mastery of disease, the larger became the symbolic and non-technical functions performed by medical technology. White coats, antiseptic environments, ambulances and insurance came to serve magical and symbolic functions influencing health. The impact of symbols, myths and rituals on health-levels is distinct from the effect of the same procedures in merely technical terms. An unnecessary or damaging shot of penicillin can still have a powerful placebo effect. As drugs become more effective, their symbolic side-effects have become overwhelmingly health-denying. In other words, the traditional white medical magic which supported the patient's own efforts has today turned black. Instead of mobilizing the patient's self-healing powers, modern medical magic turns the patient into a limp and mystified voyeur.

All rituals have a fundamental common characteristic: they increase tolerance for cognitive dissonance. Those who participate in a ritual become capable of combining an unrealistic expectation with an undesirable reality.[100] For instance, people

manipulative, somewhat impersonal ad-hoc relationship between a healer who sets the stage and specific individuals who will profit from the participation in the ritual which he conducts.

[100] GLUCKMAN, Max. *Politics, law and ritual in tribal society.* Aldine, 1965. TURNER, Victor M. *The ritual process. Structure and anti-structure.* London, Penguin Books, 1969.

who regularly and for long periods attend the ritual of schooling tend to accept the social myth that the nation-state provides equal chances to its citizens, while at the same time they learn at each moment to which precise class of citizens they belong. The more schools there are in a society, the more people will somehow come to believe in progress, even though the main effect of school has been shown to be the production of drop-outs as a majority.[101] In a similar way, the rituals of medical care will make people believe that their health is served by treatment, even though the coping ability of most people in fact declines as a result.

I happened to be in both Rio de Janeiro and Lima when Dr. Christian Barnard was touring there. In both cities he was able to fill the major football stadium twice in one day with crowds who hysterically acclaimed his macabre ability to ex-change human hearts. Medical miracle treatments have world-wide impact, their alienating effect reaching people who have no chance of access to a neighbourhood clinic, much less to a hos-pital. It provides them with an abstract assurance that 'science' is making 'progress' from which one day they too will profit. Shortly afterwards I saw well-documented evidence proving that the Brazilian police have so far been the first to use life-extending equipment and techniques in the torture chamber. Inevitably, when care or healing are transferred to organizations or machines, therapy becomes a death-centred ritual.

It would be an insult to the medicine man to call him an ancestor of the modern physician. He is in fact the ancestor of all our modern professionals. He combined and transcended functions that are now perceived to be technical, religious, legal and magic. We have lost the term to designate such a complex personage.[102]

Modern societies are deluded into believing that jobs can be specialized at will. Professionals tend to act as if the results of their actions could be limited to those having an operationally verifiable effect. Doctors heal, teachers teach, engineers trans-

[101] ILLICH, Ivan. Ritualization of progress, in: *Deschooling society*, London, Calder & Boyars, 1971, pp. 34–51.
[102] ACKERKNECHT, Erwin H. *Problems of primitive medicine*, in: Bulletin of the History of Medicine, XI, 1942, pp. 503–521.

port people and things. Economists provide a more unitary explanation for the actions of specialists by dealing with all of them as 'producers'. They have imposed on members of the liberal professions an awareness of being a kind of 'worker', often against their own will. Sociologists, however, have so far not succeeded in making these same professionals equally aware of the common ritual and magical function they serve. Just as all workers contribute to the growth of GNP, all specialists generate and sustain the delusion of progress.

Whether contemporary doctors intend to or not, they perform as priests, magicians and agents of the political establishment. When a doctor removes the adenoids of a child, he separates it for a while from its parents, exposes it to technicians who use a foreign technical language, instils in it a sense that its body may be invaded by strangers for reasons they alone know, and makes it proud to live in a country where social security pays for such medical initiations to life.[103]

When doctors set up shop outside the temple in Greece, India or China, they began to claim a rational power over sickness and left the miracle cure to priests and kings. Healing powers had always been ascribed to religious and civil authorities. The caste which had an 'in' with the gods could call for their intervention in its sanctuaries. Up to the eighteenth century the King of England imposed his hands every year upon some of those whom physicians had been unable to cure. The epileptics whose ills resisted His Majesty took recourse to the healing power flowing from the touch of the executioner.[104] The hand that wielded the knife had the power to exorcise not only the enemy but also disease. Today the medical establishment has reclaimed the right to perform miracle cures. Our contemporary medicine men

[103] 90% to 95% of all tonsillectomies performed in the U.S. are unnecessary, and yet 20 to 30% of all children undergo the operation. One in a thousand dies directly as a consequence of the operation, 16 per thousand suffer from serious complications due to the intervention. All lose valuable immunity mechanisms. Against all an emotional aggression is performed by incarcerating them in a hospital, separating them from their parents and introducing them to dependency on the unjustified and unusually pompous cruelty of the medical establishment. See LIPTON, S. D. *On psychology of childhood tonsillectomy*, in: Psychoan. stud. child. 17 (1962), pp. 363–417. Reprinted in CIDOC *Antologia A8*. See also BRANSON, Roy. *The doctor as high priest*, in: Hastings Center Studies, 1973.

[104] DANCKERT, Werner. *Unehrliche Leute. Die verfehmten Berufe*. Bern, Francke Verlag, 1963.

insist on their authority over the patient even when the aetiology is uncertain, the prognosis unfavourable, and the therapy of an experimental nature. The promise of medical miracles is their best hedge against failure, since miracles may be hoped for, but they cannot, by definition, be counted on. In our medicalized culture physicians have thus appropriated from priests and rulers the performance of the lavish rituals by which diseases are banned. Medical 'breakthroughs' serve to recover at least a part of the medicine man's role for the modern physician. When displayed on TV, medical heroics serve as a rain-dance for millions, and as liturgies in which realistic hopes for autonomous life are transmuted into the delusions that doctors will provide for humanity an ever novel kind of health.

Patient Majorities

The unbounded multiplication of sick-roles is the sixth symptom of social iatrogenesis. People who look strange or behave oddly threaten any society until their uncommon traits have been formally named and their uncommon behaviour has been slotted into a recognized role. By being assigned a name and a role, eerie and upsetting deviants are turned into well-defined and established categories. In industrial societies the abnormal is entitled to special consumption. Medical labelling has increased the number of people with exceptional consumer status to the point where people who are free of therapy-oriented labels have become the exception.

In every society there are agents who perform the task of recognizing the nature of deviance: they decide whether the member is possessed by a ghost, ridden by a god, infected by a poison, being punished for his sin, or has become the victim of vengeance by an enemy, a witch. The agents who do this labelling may be juridical, religious, military or medical authorities; in modern societies they may also be educators, social workers or party ideologues. By labelling deviants, authority places them under the control of language and custom, and turns them from a threat into a support of the social system. Once it is stated that an epileptic is ridden by the soul of a deceased person, every fit he has confirms the theory, and any strange behaviour he exhibits proves it beyond all doubt. Labelling extends social control over the forces of nature, reducing the anxiety of society.

The definition of deviance varies from culture to culture. Each civilization makes its own diseases.[105] What is sickness in one might be crime, holiness, or sin in another. The response to the deviant also varies from culture to culture. For the same symptom a man might be expelled by being killed, exiled, exposed, incarcerated or hospitalized, or he might be entitled to special respect, to alms, or to tax money.[106] A thief might be forced to wear special clothes, to do penance, to lose his fingers or be submitted to magical or technical treatment in jail or an institution for kleptomaniacs.

By the 1950s, especially in the U.S.A., the sick-role became almost totally identified with the patient role. The sick person was exonerated from most responsibility for his sickness. He was neither held accountable for having become sick nor expected to have the ability to recover on his own. His impairment excused him from social roles and obligations and relieved him from participating in normal activities. He was cast in the role of the legitimatized deviant; his exemption from his usual responsibilities was tolerated as long as he would consider his illness as an undesirable state and would seek technical assistance from the health-care system. According to this mid-century 'model of sickness' described by Talcott Parsons, sickness imposed the obligation to submit to repair service from doctors in order to return to work at the earliest date, and the worker was declared impotent to get well on his own. By identifying the sick-role with the patient role, sickness had become industrialized.[107] The

[105] TROELS, Lund. *Gesundheit und Krankheit in der Anschauung alter Zeiten.* Leipzig, 1901. An early study of the shifting frontiers of sickness in different cultures.
[106] SIGERIST, Henry E. *Civilization and disease.* University of Chicago Press, 1970.
[107] For the history of the concept of sick-role see the following. MALINOWSKI, Bronislaw, *Magic, science and religion and other essays*, N.Y., Doubleday, Anchor, 1954 (orig. 1925), who stressed that moral and religious motives underlie the explanation of illness in all cultures. HENDERSON, Lawrence J. *Physician and patient as a social system*, in: New England Journal of Medicine, Vol. 212, 1935, pp. 819–823, was one of the first to suggest that the physician exonerates the sick from moral accountability for their illness. PARSONS, Talcott. *Illness and the role of the physician.* (orig. 1948), in: KLUCKHORN, Clide., MURRAY, Henry. eds. *Personality in nature, society and culture.* Revised edition Knopf, 1953, contains the classical formulation of the modern, almost morality-free sick-role. FOX, René, *Experiment perilous. Physicians and patients facing the unknown*, Glencoe, Ill., Free Press, 1959, studies

Parsonian 'sick-role' fits modern society only for as long as doctors acted as if treatment were usually effective, and the general public were willing to share their rosy view. The mid-century sick-role has become inadequate for describing what happens in a medical system that claims authority over people who are not yet ill, people who cannot reasonably expect to get well, and those for whom doctors have no more effective treatment than that which could be offered by their wives or their aunts.

The role of the doctor has now become blurred.[108] The health professions have come to amalgamate clinical service, public health engineering and scientific medicine. The doctor deals with clients who are simultaneously cast in several roles during every contact they have with the health establishment. They are turned into patients whom medicine tests and repairs, into administered citizens whose healthy behaviour a medical bureaucracy guides, and into guinea pigs on whom medical science constantly experiments. The Aesculapian power of conferring the sick-role has been dissolved by the pretensions of delivering universal health care. Health has ceased to be a native endowment each man is presumed to possess until proven ill, and has become the ever-distant promise to which one is entitled by virtue of social justice.

The emergence of a conglomerate health profession has rendered the patient role infinitely elastic. The doctor's certification of the sick has been replaced by the bureaucratic presumption of the health manager who arranges people according to the degree and kind of their therapeutic needs. Medical authority extended to supervised health care, early detection, preventative therapies, and increasingly the treatment of the incurable. The public recognized this new right of health professionals to inter-

---

terminal patients who have given their consent to be used as subjects for medical experiment. Notwithstanding the logical and rational explanation for their sickness that prevails around them, they too grapple with their illness in religious, cosmic and especially moral terms. ROBINSON, David, *The process of becoming ill*. London, Routledge and Kegan Paul, 1971, rejects the notion that the presentation of symptoms to the professional constitutes the recognized point at which illness starts. It is the point at which the sick turns into a patient. Most people are not patients most of the time they feel ill.

[108] CHRISTIE, Nils. *Law and medicine: the case against role blurring*, in: Law and Society Review, 5 (3), Febr. 1971, pp. 357–366. A case study of the conflict between two monopolistic professional empires.

vene in the lives of people on behalf of their own health. In a morbid society the environment is so rearranged that for most of the time most people lose their power and will for self-sufficiency, and finally cease to believe that autonomous action is feasible. Previously modern medicine had controlled only the size of the market, now this market has lost all boundaries. Unsick people came to depend on professional care for the sake of their future health. The result is a morbid society that demands universal medicalization and a medical establishment that certifies universal morbidity.[109]

In a morbid society the belief prevails that defined and diagnosed ill health is infinitely preferable to any other form of negative label. It is better than criminal or political deviance, better than laziness, better than self-chosen absence from work.[110] More and more people subconsciously know that they are sick and tired of their jobs and of their leisure passivities, but they want to be lied to and told that physical illness relieves them of social and political responsibilities. They want their doctor to act as lawyer and priest. As a lawyer, the doctor exempts the patient from his normal duties and enables him to cash in on the insurance fund he was forced to build. As a priest, the doctor becomes an accomplice for the patient creating the myth that he is an innocent victim of biological mechanisms rather than a lazy, greedy or envious deserter of a social struggle for control over the tools of production. Social life becomes a give and take of therapy: medical, psychiatric, pedagogic or geriatric. Claiming access to treatment becomes a political duty,[111] and

---

[109] The rising medical consumption is explained as a growing divergence between real and felt morbidity. As health becomes heteronomous through the individual's dependence on doctors, insecurity rises and with it the sense of morbidity. On this see DUPUY, J. P. (1974), see footnote 10.

[110] Sickness becomes associated with high living standards and high expectations. In the first six months of 1970, 5 million working days were lost in Britain due to industrial disputes. This has been exceeded in only 2 years since the general strike in 1926. In comparison, over 300 million working days were lost through absence due to certified sickness. OFFICE OF HEALTH ECONOMICS. Off sick. London, OHE, 1971.

[111] SEDGWICK, Peter. Illness—mental and otherwise. This will form part of a book by Peter Sedgwick on psycho-politics to be published by Harper & Row, in: Hastings Center Studies, Vol. 1, No. 3, 1973, pp. 19–40. Sedgwick speaks of the politicalization of medical goals and argues that without the concept of illness we shall be unable to make demands on the health service facilities of the societies we

medical certification a powerful device for social control.[112]

With the development of the therapeutic service sector of the economy, an increasing proportion of all people comes to be perceived as deviating from some desirable norm and therefore as clients who can now either be submitted to therapy to bring them closer to the established standard of health, or concentrated into some special environment built to cater to their deviance. Basaglia[113] points out that in a first stage of this process, the diseased are exempted from production. At the next stage of industrial expansion a majority comes to be defined as deviant and in need of therapy. When this happens, the distance between the sick and the healthy is again reduced. In advanced industrial societies the sick are once more recognized as possessing a certain level of productivity which would have been denied them at an earlier stage of industrialization. Now that everybody tends to be a patient in some respect, wage labour acquires therapeutic characteristics. Life-long health education, hygienic counselling, testing and maintenance become part of the factory and office routine. Therapeutic relationships infiltrate and colour all productive relations. The medicalization of industrial society reinforces its imperialistic and authoritarian character.

---

live in. 'The future belongs to illness: we are going to get more and more disease since our expectations of health are going to become more expansive and sophisticated.'

[112] KARIER, Clarence, *Testing for order and control in the Corporate Liberal State*, in: Educational Theory, Vol. 22, No. 2, Spring 1972, has shown the role which the Carnegie Foundation played in developing educational testing materials which can be used for social control in situations where the ability of schools to perform this task has broken down. According to Karier tests given outside of schools are a more powerful device for discrimination than tests given within a pedagogical situation. In the same way it can be argued that medical testing becomes an increasingly more powerful means for classification and discrimination of citizens, as the number of test results increase for which no significant treatment is feasible. Once the patient role becomes universal, medical labelling turns into a tool for total social control.

[113] BASAGLIA, Franco. *La maggioranza deviante. L'ideologia del controllo sociale totale*. Torino, Nuovo Politecnico 43, Einaudi, 1971.

3 MEDICALIZATION AS A BY-PRODUCT OF AN OVER-INDUSTRIALIZED SOCIETY

THE medicalization of life is but one aspect of the destructive dominance of industry in our society. Over-medicalization is a particularly painful example of frustrating over-production. The danger of over-expansion begins to become obvious, but recognition of the danger is limited at present to the excessive growth of those industrial agencies which transform large amounts of energy. The consequent concern with necessary limits to further growth in the goods sector of the economy distracts attention from the danger of overgrowth in the services sector. In fact, most advocates of limits to growth argue for a shift of manpower and funds from the production of hardware to education, health and other forms of welfare. If accepted, their recommendations will only aggravate the present crisis.

We live in an epoch in which learning is programmed, residence urbanized, traffic motorized, communication channelled, and where for the first time nearly one-third of all foodstuffs consumed by humanity passes through inter-regional markets. In such an over-industrialized society, people are conditioned to get things rather than to do them. They want to be taught, moved, treated or guided rather than learn, heal and find their own way. The transitive use of the verb 'healing' comes to prevail. 'Healing' ceases to be considered the activity of the sick and becomes increasingly the duty of the physician. Soon it can be turned from a personal service into the product of an agency. Over-medicalization and its unwanted by-products are thus part of a deep and general crisis that affects all our major institutions.

Schools produce education, motor vehicles produce locomotion and medicine produces clinical care. These outputs are staples that have all the characteristics of commodities. The total cost of a passenger mile, the total cost of a high school education, or the total cost of a colostomy are more or less the same whether they reach the customer on a free market or as public utilities. Their production costs can be added to or subtracted from the GNP, their scarcity measured in terms of marginal value, and their cost established in currency equivalents. They come in different quanta, hierarchically arranged, and access to the higher and more costly package usually supposes that the consumer has already obtained access to the system at a lower level. Universities are open only to high school graduates, regional hospitals to those who are referred from the community clinic, and aeroplane seats to those for whom the community also provides transport to the airport. A few people will get much more of a certain commodity than others, though all must pay for the production. The training of a Peruvian physician costs about six thousand times the median amount spent on the education of a Peruvian peasant. Once that much has been spent on one man's education, his knowledge capital will be valued and protected. His share in the international knowledge stock will entitle him to equally disproportionate amounts of international travel and medical maintenance. Industrial outputs are not only packaged and bundled; the large bundles also tend to go to the same few addresses. School education, motor transportation, and clinical care are products of a capital-intensive mode of production. Each of these products competes with a non-marketable use value which people have always enjoyed in an autonomous mode. People learn by seeing and doing; they move on their own, they heal, they take care of their health and the health of others. Most of the use values thus produced resist marketing. Most learning, locomotion or healing do not show up in the GNP. They are use values, and they are fairly evenly distributed among the general population. People learn their mother tongue, move around on their feet, produce their children and bring them up, recover the use of a broken bone and prepare the local diet, and they do all these things with more or less the same competence and enjoyment. These are all valuable though self-limiting activities, which most of the time will not and cannot be undertaken for money.[114]

114 Studying the effectiveness of pre-capitalist production: CHAYANOV, A. V. *Theory of peasant economy*. In 1966 Irwin had already demonstrated that 'productive intensity is inversely related to productive capacity'. Discussing the domestic mode of production SAHLINS, Marshall, *Stone age economics*, Aldine, Chicago 1972, says: 'For the greater part of human history, labour has been more significant than tools, the intelligent efforts of the producer more decisive than his simple equipment.' On p. 81 he discusses and quotes supporting evidence from MARX, Karl, *Grundrisse*, 1857.

In the achievement of each major social objective, these two modes of need-satisfaction complemented each other, but in our time they conflict increasingly. When most needs of most people are satisfied in a domestic or community mode of production, the gap between expectations and gratification tends to be narrow and stable. Learning, locomotion or sick care are the results of highly decentralized initiatives, of autonomous inputs and self-limiting total outputs. Under these conditions of subsistence the tools used in production determine the needs which the application of these same tools can also fulfil. People, for instance, know what they can expect when they get sick. Somebody in the village or nearby town knows all the remedies that have worked in the past, and beyond this lies the supernatural and unpredictable realm of the miracle. Until late into the 19th century, most families even in Western countries provided most of the therapy that was known. Most learning, locomotion or healing was performed by each man on his own or in his family or village setting.

Autonomous production can be supplemented by industrial outputs. It can be rendered both more effective and more decentralized by using such industrially made tools as bicycles, books or antibiotics. But it can also be hampered, devalued and blocked by a rearrangement of society totally in favour of industry. Such a rearrangement has two sides: people are trained for consumption rather than for action, and at the same time their range of action is narrowed. The structure of the tool alienates the workman from his labour. Trained commuters are frustrated to find their bicycles pushed off the road, and trained patients to find grandmother's remedies available only on prescription. Wage-labour and client-relationships expand while autonomous production and gift-relationships wither.[115]

Achieving social objectives effectively depends on the degree to which these two modes of production supplement or hamper each other. Effectively coming to know a given physical and social environment and controlling it depends on people's education and on their opportunity and motivation to learn on their own. Effective traffic depends on the ability of people to get where they must go quickly and conveniently. Effective sick care depends on the degree to which pain and dysfunction are made tolerable and

[115] SAHLINS, Marshall. ibid. The spirit of the gift, pp. 149 ff, see also footnote 114.

recovery is enhanced. The effective satisfaction of these needs must be clearly distinguished from the efficiency with which industrial products are made and marketed. The criteria by which effective need satisfaction can be evaluated do not match the measurements used to evaluate the production and marketing of industrial goods.

When the industrial mode of production expands within a society, the measurements applied to its growth tend to neglect the values produced by the autonomous mode.[116] Literacy statistics give the number of people who have been serially taught in school, not of those who have learned to read from the teacher or on their own, much less of those who actually read for enjoyment. People on Mexican buses illustrate the point. Professionals do not ride them. Some who ride and read are students. But most adults who read with single-minded attention stick their noses into a unique kind of book or pamphlet: an instructive and political comic like *Supermachos* or *Agachados*, or one of a more sentimental kind. Overwhelmingly these are people who have either not been to school or have not finished the five years of compulsory schooling. On the statistical tables they show up as illiterates. Statistics do not indicate who learns more and who learns less. In the same way, traffic statistics give passenger miles. They sometimes give them by residence, income, size of vehicle and age. But traffic statistics do not tell who now walks more and who walks less; they do not tell us who is the slave and who is the lord of traffic.

Since measurements disregard the contributions made by the autonomous mode towards the total effectiveness with which any major social goal will be achieved, they cannot indicate if this total effectiveness is increasing or decreasing. Much less can technical measurements indicate who are the beneficiaries and who are the losers from industrial growth. Who are the few who get more and can do more, and who fall into the majority whose marginal access to industrial products is compounded by their loss of autonomous effectiveness.[117]

[116] These measurements were created ad-hoc during the last generation. See SPENGLER, Joseph. *Quantification in economics: its history*, in: LERNER, Daniel, ed., *Quantity and Quality*. The Hayden Colloquium on Scientific Method and Concept. Free Press, 1959, pp. 129–211.

[117] On the inefficient society see also: SCHWARTZ, Eugene S., *Overskill; the decline of technology in modern civilization*. Chicago, Quadrangle Books, 1971.

Logically, those most hurt are not the poorest in monetary terms. The poor in Mexico or India have learned to survive by making do on their own, and they can survive because their environment does not yet impede them from fending for themselves. Those most hurt are certain types of consumers for whom the U.S. elderly can serve as a paradigm. They have been trained to experience urgent needs which no level of relative privilege can possibly satisfy; at the same time their ability to take care of themselves has withered, and social arrangements allowing such autonomy have practically disappeared. They are examples of modern poverty created by industrial overgrowth.

The elderly in the U.S. are only an extreme example of suffering promoted by high cost deprivation. Having learned to consider old age akin to disease, they develop unlimited economic needs paying for interminable therapies which are usually ineffective, frequently demeaning and painful, and which most often call for recovery in a special milieu.

Five features of industrially modernized poverty appear as caricatures in the pampered slums of rich men's retirement: first, the incidence of chronic diseases increase as fewer people die in their youth; second, more people suffer clinical damage from health measures; third, medical services grow more slowly than the spread and urgency of demand; fourth, people find fewer resources in their environment and culture which can help them to come to terms with their suffering and they are therefore forced to depend on medical services for a wider range of trivia; and fifth, people have lost the ability to come to terms with impairment or pain and have become dependent on the management of every 'discomfort' by specialized servicemen. The cumulative result of over-expansion in the health care industry has thwarted the power of people to cope with challenges and to adapt to change in their bodies or change in the environment. This loss of autonomy is further reinforced by a political prejudice. The politics of health consistently place the improvement of medical care above those factors which would improve and equalize ability for modern self-care.

Political prejudice concentrates the criticism of today's radicals on five shortcomings of the medical industry. First, production of remedies and services has become self-serving. Consumer lobbies 'ought' to force doctors to improve their service. Second, the delivery of remedies and the access to services is unequal and arbitrary; it either depends on the patient's money and rank, or on a social prejudice in favour of treating heart disease rather than hunger. The nationalization of all services 'ought' to control the hidden hand of the clinic. Third, the organization of the medical guild perpetuates inefficiency and privilege and imposes the prejudice of one school of doctors on an entire society. This latter is a fourth shortcoming which like the previous ones 'ought' to be remedied by more lay-participation in the selection of candidates for medical schools and in the making of medical policy. Finally, the main concern of present medicine is sick individuals rather than the health of populations. More health engineering is almost always proposed. The political remedies for these shortcomings have one thing in common: they tend to reinforce further medicalization. Only a substantial reduction in total medical outputs could foster autonomy in health and in sick care, and thereby make it effective.

4 FUTILE POLITICAL COUNTER-MEASURES

Consumer Protection for Addicts

PEOPLE have become aware of their dependence on the medical industry but believe that it is irreversible. As in transportation or housing, they speak of the need for consumer protection and feel that political power can check the high-handedness of medical producers. But the sad truth is that neither control of cost or quality guarantee that health will be served by the activity of doctors.

When consumers band together to force General Motors to sell an acceptable car, they feel competent to look under the hood and they have criteria for estimating the cost of improvements. When they band together to get better medical care, they are in a different situation. They believe mistakenly that they are not competent to decide what ought to be done for their bowels, and blindly entrust themselves to the doctor for this service.

Titmuss[118] has summed up the difficulty of cost-benefit accounting in medicine, especially at a time when medical care is losing the characteristics it used to possess when it consisted almost wholly of the personal doctor-patient relationship. Medical care is uncertain and unpredictable; many consumers do not desire it, do not know that they need it, and cannot know in advance what it would cost them. They cannot learn from experience. They must rely on the supplier to tell them if they have been well served, and cannot return the service to the seller or have it repaired. Medical services are not advertised as are other goods, and the producer discourages comparison. Once he has purchased, a consumer cannot change his mind in mid-treatment. The medical producer has the power to select his consumers and to market some products which will be forced on the consumer, if need be, by the intervention of the police: the

[118] TITMUSS, Richard M. *The culture of medical care and consumer behaviour,* in: POINTER, F. N. L. ed. *Medicine and Culture.* 1969, chap. 8, pp. 129–135.

producers can even sell forcible internment for the disabled and asylums for the mentally retarded.

The normal consumer of medical care just does not and cannot exist. Nobody can know how much health care will be worth to him in money or in pain. In addition, nobody can know if the most advantageous form of health care is best purchased from medical producers, travel bureaux, or by renouncing work on the nightshift. The economics of health is a curious discipline, somewhat in the tradition of the theology of indulgences which flourished before Luther. You can count what the friars collect, you can look at the temples they build, you can take part in the liturgies they indulge in, but you can only guess what the traffic in amnesties for purgatory does to the soul after death. Models developed to account for the rising willingness of tax-payers to foot rising medical bills provide similar scholastic guesswork about the new world-spanning church of medicine. To give an example: it is possible to view health as a durable capital stock used to produce an output called 'healthy time'.[119] Individuals inherit an initial stock which can be increased by investment in health capitalization: through the acquisition of medical care, or through good diet and housing. 'Healthy time' is an article in demand for two reasons: as a consumption commodity it directly enters into the individual's utility function; besides, people usually would rather be healthy than sick. It also enters into the market as an investment commodity. In this function, 'healthy time' determines the amount of time an individual can spend on work and on play, on earning and on recreation. The individual's 'healthy time' can thus be viewed as a decisive indicator of his value to the community as a producer.[120] This is simply saying in a roundabout way what every Mexican brick-

[119] GROSSMAN, Michael. *On the concept of health capital and the demand for health*, in: Journal of Political Economy, 80, March–April, 1972. pp. 223–255.

[120] For other 'theologies' see BERKOWITZ, Monroe. JOHNSON, William G. *Towards an economics of disability: the magnitude and structure of transfer and medical costs*, in: Journal of Human Resources, 5, Summer, 1970, pp. 271–297. Berkowitz attempts to put a dollar-value on the economic losses sustained from the disability of the working man in the U.S. These include medical costs for treating the disabled, disability payments and pensions, and the forfeiture of goods and services not produced as a result of these disabilities. DOWIE, J. A. *Valueing the benefit of health improvement*, in: Australian Economic Papers, 9, June, 1970, pp. 21–24, gives a conceptual re-formulation of benefits derived from health improvements and death prevention.

layer knows: only on days when he is healthy enough to work can he bring beans and tortillas to his children and have a tequila with his friends. But this obvious value of health allows neither the bricklayer nor the health economist[121] to evaluate the role which medical expenditures play in keeping him at work.

People in modern societies believe that they depend on the medical industry, but they do not know for what purpose. Different political approaches have been used to legitimatize the tax-supported output of doctors. Socialist nations assume the financing of all care and leave it to the medical profession to define what is needed, how it must be done, who may do it, what it should cost, and also who shall get it. Some other nations intervene with laws and incentives in the organization of their health care systems. Only the U.S. launched a national legislative programme to assure the quality of care offered on the 'free market' and has left it entirely to the representatives of the medical profession to determine what shall be considered good care.

In late 1973 President Nixon signed Public Law 92–603 establishing mandatory cost and quality controls (by Professional Standard Review Organizations) for the tax-supported sector of the medical industry, which since 1970 has been second in size only to the military-industrial complex. Harsh financial sanctions threaten physicians if they refuse to open their files to government inspectors searching for evidence of over-utilization of hospitals, fraud or deficient treatment. The law requires the medical profession to establish guidelines for the diagnosis and treatment of a long list of injuries, illnesses and health conditions. This is the world's most costly programme for the medicalization of health-production by means of legislated consumer protection. The new law guarantees the quality of a commodity. It does not question if its delivery is related to the health of the people.[122]

Attempts to exercise rational political control over the production of contemporary medicine have consistently failed. The

[121] ENTERLINE, Philip E. *Social causes of sick absence*, in: Archives of Environmental Health, 12, April, 1966, p. 467.
[122] WELCH, Claude, *PSRO's—pros and cons*, in: The New England Journal of Medicine, Vol. 290, 1974, p. 1319 ff. *Idem.*, Vol. 289, 1973, p. 291 and pps. 1045–1046.

reason lies in the nature of the product now conceived of as 'medicine'. This product is a package made up of chemicals, apparatus, buildings and specialists and delivered as medicine to the client. The purveyor rather than his clients or political boss defines the size of the package. The patient is reduced to an object being repaired; he is no longer a subject being helped to heal. If he is allowed to participate in the repair process, he acts as the last apprentice in a hierarchy of repairmen.[123] Usually he is not even trusted to take a pill without getting it from a nurse. The medical profession has cornered the prerogative of administering most applications of modern science to health care. The argument that institutional health care (remedial or preventative) after a certain point ceases to correlate with any further 'gains' in health can be misused for transforming clients hooked to doctors into clients of some other service hegemony. The consumer is encouraged to ask himself where health services should end and where other social services would contribute more decisively to his health status or to that of his group.[124] What begins as consumer protection quickly turns into a crusade to transform independent people into clients at all cost. Any kind of dependence turns into an obstacle to autonomous mutual care, coping, adapting and healing and, what is worse, into a device by which people are stopped from transforming the conditions at work and at home which do make them sick. Control over the production side of the medical complex can work towards better health only if it leads to a very sizeable reduction of its total output, rather than simply to technical improvements in the wares which are offered.

Egalitarian Access to Torts

As a political issue health usually translates into equitable

[123] DEWAR, Tom. *Some notes on the professionalization of the client.* Cuernavaca, CIDOC, 1973. I/V 73/37. Licensing is the key to medical power. Doctors can set standards for their own training, behaviour, and performance. They can set standards for the training of all those who assist them, for the quality of all organizations or devices they use. The unlimited power of licensing thus removes all limits to medical power. How this works in the American Medical Association has been well described by RAYACK, Elton. *Professional power and American medicine: the economics of the American Medical Association.* Cleveland, World Publishing Co., 1967.

[124] HAGGERTY, Robert J. *The boundaries of health care,* in: The Pharos, July, 1972, pp. 106–111.

care.[125] Political parties coin the desire for health into the design of medical facilities. They do not question what kind of things the medical system produces but insist that their constituents have a right to those things that are produced for the rich. Any intimation that the total amount earmarked for health services ought to be reduced immediately evokes the idea that the poor would be the first to suffer. This objection to control over the size of the medical industry can be dealt with only if it turns out that the poor and the rich are equally hurt by medical over-production. Two distinct kinds of claims tend to be made by politicians: first, that poor people get less medical care than the rich; and second, that poor people are less healthy and need more. Both claims warrant analysis.

In most countries the poor have less access to medical services than the rich. In all Latin American countries except Cuba, the poorest fifth are those among whom only one child in forty will finish the five years of compulsory schooling, and about the same proportion of the population will receive treatment in a hospital when sick. The rich are the 3% made up of college graduates, their families, labour leaders, and higher officials of all political parties. These receive treatment from the doctors of their choice, almost all of whom come from their own ranks and have been trained to international standards on government grants.[126]

Notwithstanding unequal access to care by physicians, it would be wrong to say that access to medical service always correlates with personal income. In Mexico, 3% of the population has

[125] HIRSHFIELD, Daniel S. *The lost reform: the campaign for compulsory health insurance in the United States from 1932 to 1943.* Cambridge, Harvard Univ. Press, 1970, provides evidence that, at least in the U.S.A. and for the last sixty years, the public policy discussion about health-care has at no moment transcended the industrial paradigm of medicine as an engineering enterprise. This book has an excellent bibliography.

[126] 'It is my belief that the tendency of Government health services in Latin America to concentrate on medical care has been very harmful. In Venezuela for instance, the annual cost of a hospital bed is about ten times the average income in the country.' GABALDON, Arnoldo. *Health services and socio-economic development in Latin America*, in: The Lancet, April 12, 1969, pp. 739–744. See also NAVARRO, Vicente. *The under-development of health or the health of under-development, an analysis of the distribution of human resources in Latin America.* Johns Hopkins University. Paper based on presentation at Pan American Conference of Health Manpower Planning, Ottawa, Canada, September 10–14, 1973.

access to a social security system which holds a world record in combining personal care with professional excellence. This fortunate group is made up of government employees who receive truly equal treatment, whether they are ministers or office boys.

This minority can count on high quality care because they are part of a demonstration model. The surgeons who operate on them measure up to the standards of their colleagues in Texas. The newspapers can, accordingly, inform the schoolmaster in a remote village that Mexican surgery is even better endowed than hospitals in Chicago. When high-level officials are hospitalized, they may be put out because for the first time in their lives they sleep next to a workman, but they are also proud of the high level of democratic commitment their nation shows in providing the same for boss and custodian. Both kinds of patient tend to overlook that they are both privileged exploiters. To provide them with beds, equipment, administration, and technical care, one-third of the health care budget of the entire country must be allotted to this tiny minority. To give all of the poor equal access to medicine of uniform quality, most of the present activities of the health professions would have to be discontinued.

The U.S. ranks seventeenth amongst the nations of the world in infant mortality. It is generally assumed that this rank is related to social and political factors, especially to an infant mortality rate among the poorest group which is much higher than the median. One-fifth of the American people are considered economically disadvantaged, and within this group the rate of infant mortality exceeds some of the so-called underdeveloped countries in Africa and Asia. A common explanation is that the poor have less money to spend on the health package. Contrary to a widely held belief, this is not generally true. Use of the physician's services in the U.S. is not directly related to income. Low-income families do not receive less but more medical care than the income group immediately above them.[127] These low-income middle Americans are too poor to pay doctors out of their own pockets and too rich for access to those special funds set aside for the certified poor. The factor responsible for the high rate of infant mortality even among the poorest in the U.S. is only to a marginal degree a lag in therapeutic consumption.

[127] GLAZER, Nathan. *Paradoxes of health care*, in: The Public Interest, pp. 62–77.

A more likely explanation is that the mode of U.S. therapeutic consumption lies above the level at which more expenditure can increase well-being. By the time a U.S. child has survived his post-natal care, from which he is less and less able to escape no matter how poor or hungry, he has already been hurt not only by his environment but also by his collision with an over-equipped medical system.[128]

Differences in infant mortality rates between different social groups must now be imputed to environmental and cultural factors which are becoming more significant prognostic indicators than access to medical care.[129] Over-eating, tension, travel, over-medication and other factors associated with high income shorten the life of the rich adult, while crowding, pollution, crime, discrimination and second-rate contact with the health system are more threatening to the life of the poor child. Extra therapy of the kind now offered adds to the total negative impact which a poor environment has on the health of the poor. Less access to the present health system would, contrary to political rhetoric, benefit the poor.

In a society in which medical services are available only through government agencies, the elimination of iatrogenic interventions presents no political dilemma, at least in theory. The government can protect all equally. When it is recognized that any medical performance has no results, or negative results, the government can simply decide to discontinue the procedure. In countries that do not have central financing, planning and control of health services, the same recognition creates a major political dilemma. Even if costly health services are denied tax money, their elimination cannot be effected nor will their

[128] BIRCH, Herbert T., GUSSOW, Joan Dye. *Disadvantaged children: health, nutrition and school failure*, N.Y., Harcourt, Brace and World, 1970. Though the authors believe in the value of more medical care for the poor, the non-treatment related factors which discriminate against the health of poor children are indicated as being by far the most important.

[129] The relationship of mortality to both medical care and environmental variables is examined in a regression analysis by AUSTER, Richard et al. *The production of health, an exploratory study*, in: Journal of Human Res. 4, Fall 1969, pp. 411–436. If education and medical care are controlled, high income is associated with high mortality. This probably reflects unfavourable diets, lack of exercise and psychological tension in the richer groups. Adverse factors associated with the growth of income may be nullifying the beneficial effects of an increase in the quantity and quality of medical care.

73

prestige value diminish. Undeniably these services yield low benefits relative to their cost, they represent a positive danger to the well-being of the client, and their damaging effects can spill over into the community. It is, however, true that the poor will be spared disappointments and direct damages and also, since there will be fewer interventions, some of the communal spill-over effect. Considering only the technical functions of medicine, it seems reasonable to oppose government spending which has the purpose of equalizing access to potentially damaging medical performances. But the matter is not that simple, because medicine is not only a technical service, but also a status symbol. Symbolic satisfaction has become a major purpose of medical expenditures and provides recognized rewards. People have come to believe that hospitalization, tests, drugs and psycho-therapy are a privilege and that the best proof that this privilege is desirable are the huge amounts spent by those who can afford it. In a free society, so long as the current prejudice in favour of medicalization prevails, government will be forced to allocate resources according to public demand, even if they do not effectively accomplish what the public desires. Under these circumstances, the political control of health delivery services cannot but strengthen the hand of their producers.

The more people come to depend on access to modern service institutions, the more important it seems to determine what constitutes equitable access. Is equity realized when equal numbers of dollars are available for the education of rich and poor? Or is it necessary that these dollars be actually spent equally? Or does equity require that the poor get the same 'education' though much more will have to be spent on their account to achieve equal results? This battle of equity versus equality in the access to institutional care, which has already been waged in the field of education, is now being initiated in the field of medical care.[130] Whoever wins, the school and medical systems will be strengthened because the issue is not education and health but equal access to professional care, illusions and torts.

Public control of a growth-oriented medical industrial complex will reinforce its health-denying expansion. We have already seen

[130] FEIN, Rashi. *On achieving access and equity in health care*, in: Milbank Memorial Fund Quarterly, Oct., 1972, Vol. 50:34.

that this paradoxical effect will follow public controls if these focus on engineering and delivery. The industry's monopoly over health care must increase as long as the public organizes its energies to distribute 'better' goods more equitably. Only a negative growth rate of the medical complex could promote equal access to healthy care.

Public Control over the Medical Mafia

A third kind of public policy, namely the attempt to control the internal organization of the medical profession, has equally health-denying effects.

I have avoided blaming either self-serving production or un-equal service on the greed of doctors. Practice for personal gain explains neither. Both problems persist whether doctors themselves set their fees, fees are set for doctors, or all doctors are made into civil servants. Fundamentally, social iatrogenesis is not due to the individual behaviour of any number of doctors but to the radical monopoly the profession as such has attained.

It is true that in some countries many doctors become very rich. This is a symptom of economic exploitation, but not an explanation for the unhealthy effects of medical practice. Unfortunately, many critics of U.S. or French medicine believe that if only doctors were put on salaries, a major step would have been made towards healthier practice. The contrary might be true: by closing the gap between the income of interns and full practitioners, and by setting a ceiling on their earnings, the whole of a publicly regulated medical profession could well gain in cohesion and prestige and claim a larger proportion of national wealth to en-large its ranks and increase its power. The existence of a few charlatans or racketeers has always served the credibility of the medical guild: by denouncing their misbehaviour, the typical practitioner could legitimatize the abuses inherent in his ordinary practice. In the same way, exploitation by individual doctors now blinds people to the exploitation of the commonweal by the health profession as a whole. Public control over the private enrichment of a few individuals could easily become a powerful device for legitimatizing an even more intensive medicalization of life.

Besides objecting to private enrichment, the general public

75

questions the hierarchical organization of medical care. Doctors are thought to lord it over health care and reduce their assistants to ancillary roles. But most proposed alternatives tighten the integration of the medical care industry and 'increase efficiency by upward mobility of personnel and downward assignment of responsibility'.[131] The argument that doctors now do what nurses could do better leads to a demand for more types of para-professionals[132] and multiplies the professional organizations, congresses and unions. An increase of para-professionals decreases what people may do for each other and for themselves.

U.S. prescribing doctors, competent surgeons, and independent pharmacists worked independently side-by-side until about a hundred years ago.[133] The first was a kind of gentleman, the second an artisan, and the third a merchant. Some sixty years ago, the university-trained doctor imposed his authority. With his advent the independent practice of the pharmacist, midwife, bone-setter and tooth-puller, as well as first-aid and grandmother's self-care began to decline. The number of people with health skills decreased. More medical corps men for Harlem, more feldschers for Baku or more specialized training and supervision for Chinese barefoot doctors, far from being steps towards the deprofessionalization of health care, are policies equivalent to more power to the barons rather than to the people.[134]

As long as doctors alone decide what constitutes good service,

[131] RUSHMER, Robert F. *Medical engineering: projections for health care delivery.* N.Y., Academic Press, 1972. Besides, a mere reorganization of hierarchies might increase exploitation rather than decrease it.

[132] GISH, Oscar, editor. *Health, manpower and the medical auxiliary. Some notes and an annotated bibliography.* Intermediate Technology Development Group, London, 1971.

[133] SHYROCK, Richard Harrison. *Medicine and society in America: 1660–1860.* Ithaca, N.Y., Great Seal Books, 1962.

[134] Nursing personnel is becoming scarce. Poor salaries, growing disdain for servant and housekeeping roles, an increase in the number of chronic patients (and consequent growing tedium in their care) and new opportunities for women in other fields, all contribute to a manpower crisis. In England 70% of all low-level hospital personnel comes from overseas. Similar rates prevail in Germany and France, and in the U.S. for Puerto Rican, Mexican and Black employees. The creation of new ranks, titles, curricula, roles and specialities is a doubtfully effective remedy. The hospital only reflects the labour economy of a high-technology society: specialization on the top, a new sub-proletariat at the bottom and progressive professionalization of the client. For the current crisis in the U.S. nursing profession see NATIONAL COMMISSION FOR THE STUDY OF NURSING AND NURSING EDUCATION. *An abstract for action.* N.Y., McGraw-Hill, 1970.

they cannot be told what medical services will cost: at best they can be told how much the public is willing to grant them as personal income. As long as doctors decide who may give good service, at best they can be told to assign a quota of black doctors and encourage Puerto Ricans in the United States or Uzbekhs in Russia to become physiotherapists: in the process such therapy will become more of a professional service and less of a general skill.[135]

In fifteen years the number of specialties recognized by the American Medical Association has more than doubled and now includes sixty-seven fields. Within each field a fiefdom develops, with recognized nurses, technicians, journals, congresses, and sometimes organized groups of patients pressing for more public funds. The cost of co-ordinating the treatment of the same patient by several specialists grows exponentially with each added competence involved in the process, and so does the risk of mistakes and the probability of damage due to the unexpected synergy of different therapies. Each citizen tends to be placed into a patient relationship with each of several specialists. The number of patient relationships outgrows the number of people. As long as the public bows to the professional monopoly in assigning the sick role, it cannot control the multiplication of patients.

Tax Support to All Medical Sects

The medical profession has largely ceased to pursue the goals of an association of artisans who apply tradition, expertise, learning and intuition, and has come to play a role formerly reserved to the priesthood, using scientific principles as its theology and technologists as its acolytes. Physicians are no longer concerned with the practical art of healing the curable, but with the salvation of mankind from the shackles of illness, impairment, and even the necessity of death. The medical profession has ceased to be a true guild, with craftsmen applying rules established to guide the masters of a practical art for the benefit of real sick persons. It has become an orthodox party of bureaucratic administrators who

[135] DAVIS, K. *The role of technology demand and labour markets in the determination of hospital costs.* Communication à la Conférence sur l'Economie de la Santé et des Soins Médicaux, Tokyo, April 1973, mimeo.

apply scientific principles and methods to whole categories of medical cases. In other words, scientific medicine has taken over the clinic.[136] For the 'scientific' doctor, medicine is a science, and each treatment is one more repetition of an experiment with a statistically defined probability of success. As in any operation that constitutes a genuine application of science, failure is said to be due to some sort of ignorance: the lack of scientific knowledge about the laws that apply in the particular experimental situation, the lack of personal competence in the application of methods and principles on the part of the experimenter, or else his inability to control that elusive variable which is the patient. The better the patient is controlled, the more predictable the outcome in such medicine.

Medical science applied by medical scientists is expected to provide the correct treatment, regardless of whether its results are a cure, death, or no reaction on the part of the patient. It is legitimatized by statistical tables, which predict mathematically all three results. Its practitioners corporately constitute a bureaucracy, not a guild. In contrast, the individual doctor owes nature and the patient as much gratitude as the patient owes him if he has been successful in the use of his art. The practitioners of this art could somehow control each other and protect the public by forming a guild, albeit the most liberal one.

At present, the medical corps retains the power to define health and to determine which methods of care deserve public financing. It rules against heretical opinions and can deprive those who apply them of public support, if not of the right to practise. Since the beginning of the century, the medical corps has been an established church. Another kind of radical politics tries to mount an attack against this bureaucratically-enforced ideology.

The legal actions proposed to break this quasi-ecclesiastical monopoly have historical precedents. Other churches have been disestablished in the past. Four models of disestablishment have been tried. The first favours tradition. It deprives the Pope of secular assistance when he has fulminated against a heretic.

---

[136] The technocrats of medicine tend to promote the interest of science rather than the needs of society. The argument is strongly formulated by LEACH, Gerald. *The biocrats: implications of medical progress.* New York, McGraw-Hill, 1970; Baltimore, Penguin Books, revised ed., 1972.

Neither his power to claim tax money nor his right to determine marriage legislation are touched. In many modern countries this level of liberality has not yet been reached in the field of medicine. People still go to jail if, measured by medical dogma, they are branded as quacks. The second form of disestablishment grants equal privileges to two or more churches. Catholics and Lutherans have equal rights to tax collection in the German Federal Republic. In the medical field not only established professionals but also homeopaths and chiropractors would get a slice of the tax cake. A third is the U.S. model of a rigid separation of Church and State. Disestablishment in this case is a meticulous denial of all direct support through tax funds without any denial of or suspicion against the goals pursued by the Church. In this model churches are seen as probably necessary, and certainly inevitable, institutions. The disestablishment of medicine on this model would be achieved if no funds were ever used for the direct support of a medical institution. A fourth form of disestablishment is toleration of churches on the Russian model: churches are seen as unhealthy; they are supervised and taxed. Nobody in his right mind would propose this model for the disestablishment of medical care institutions.

Proposals which aim to provide more legal equality to alternative medical models all aim in some way at the disestablishment of the medical 'church'. They tend to fall into the second, equal privileges, model. The net effect of this kind of therapeutic pluralism might easily be more corporate medicine. Acupuncturists, Ayurveds, homeopaths, and witches can be assigned departments in a world-wide hospital for life-long patients. In a therapy-oriented society, all kinds of Aesculapians[137] can share in the monopoly of assigning the sick role, but the more different professional cliques can exempt the sick from their normal obligations, the less people on their own define how they wish to be known and treated. Unless the disestablishment of

[137] According to SIEGLER, Miriam and OSMOND, Humphry. *Aesculapian authority*, in: Hastings Center Studies, Vol. 1, No. 2, 1973, pp. 41–52, Aesculapian authority was first mentioned in PATERSON, T. T. *Notes on Aesculapian authority*, unpublished manuscript, 1957. The Aesculapian authority constitutes a bundle of three roles: sapiential authority to advise, instruct and direct; moral authority which makes medical actions the right thing, and not just something good, and charismatic authority by which the doctor can appeal to some supreme power, and which often outranks the patient's conscience and the *raison d'état*.

the medical corps leads to more access by the citizen to self-cure, it will reinforce rather than reduce sickening medicalization.

Paracelus teaches how to reduce pain by treating the lesion with herbs, and the acupuncturist how to lessen pain with needles. The Ayurved makes one responsible for all sickness, shows how to forget pain and sickness, and teaches that for the love of God you should bear both. Contemporary medicine suffers from one delusion that distinguishes it from all predecessors. It assumes that all ills ought to be treated, whatever the predictable outcome. Unfortunately, this therapeutic mania is infectious and has crippled the traditional art of sick care. The scope of professional activities has become so wide that licensing has become meaningless and certainly useless for any self-control by the professions.

The Chinese were the first to 'establish' their medicine, creating imperial colleges for its teaching and imperial certification to verify, every five years, whether the practitioner still kept up his knowledge. The mandarins were the first to attempt to prolong life by scientifically concocted elixirs. For centuries they preserved valuable records about their poisonous effects while trying them again and again. The new medical mandarins of China are the first to combine the medical art of traditional healers with an industrial enterprise aimed at indefinite progress in technological medicine. It remains to be seen how long traditional remedies will remain in use although incorporated in a therapy-oriented system.

Health care is now costly and unevenly distributed, but multiplying health professionals would only increase symptoms, therapies and demands. The control by doctors over the production of medical goods renders them scarce. Increased budgets, more rational production, more public controls over distribution, the reduction of medical privileges, and a return from scientific to clinical medicine could decrease costs, render access more equitable, and treatment more effective. But there is also a great advantage to the present limitations. Limited medical benefits also mean limited iatrogenic by-products. If outputs were to be increased, goals more rationally controlled, and distribution of access more equitable, the present system could deepen its sickening effect and decrease the coverage for self-care.

Engineering for a Plastic Womb

So far I have dealt with four categories of criticism directed at the institutional structure of the medical-industrial complex. Each gives rise to a specific kind of political demand, and all of them become reinforcements for the dependence of people on medical bureaucracies because they deal with health care as a form of therapeutic planning and engineering.[138] They indicate strategies for surgical, chemical, and behavioural intervention in the lives of sick people or people threatened with sickness. A fifth category of criticism rejects these objectives. Without relinquishing the view of medicine as an engineering endeavour, these critics assert that medical strategies fail because they concentrate too much effort on sickness and too little on changing the environment that makes people sick.

Most research on alternatives to clinical intervention is directed towards programme engineering for the professional systems of man's social, psychological and physical environment. 'Non-health-service health determinants' are largely concerned with planned intervention on the milieu.[139] Therapeutic engineers shift the thrust of their interventions from the potential or actual patient towards the larger system of which he is an imagined

[138] DUNAYE, Thomas M. *Health planning: a bibliography of basic readings*, Council of Planning Librarians: Exch. Bibliography, 1968, mimeo and reproduced in CIDOC *Antologia A2*, says: 'So extensive is the literature of source materials on the subject of health planning that to provide a complete bibliography has become an elephantine problem. This difficulty has been partially overcome by the assembly of separate bibliographies ... many of which are included ... [in this] ... unified body of basic readings useful to the ... newcomer to the field. See also SANGSTER, R. P. *Ecology, a selected bibliography*. Council of Planning Librarians; Exchange Bibliography. January 1971.

[139] As an example of this approach see: LERNER, Monroe., BRENNER, Harvey, CASSEL, John., et al. *The non-health services' determinants of health levels: conceptualization and public policy implications*. Report of a sub-committee under the Carnegie Grant to the Medical Sociology Section, American Sociological Association, August 29, 1973, mimeo. Faced with the need to identify the limits of its field, the committee came to some useful conclusions: 1. it will deal with factors affecting health levels, or perceived as doing so; not with concepts, measurements of health levels or externalities of health for improvement of socio-cultural levels; 2. it will deal with factors that affect populations at risk selectively; 3. with the prevention, maintenance, adaptation to chronic illness and disability, but only so long as these are not perceived as 'health services'; 4. it will also deal with the unintended ill-health caused by contact with the system for the delivery of personal health.

part. Instead of manipulating the sick, they re-design the environment to ensure a healthier population.[140]

Health care, as environmental hygienic engineering, works within categories different from those of the clinical scientist. Its focus is human survival rather than disease; the impact of stress on populations rather than the impact of specific agents on individuals; the relationship of the human niche in the cosmos to the species with which it has evolved rather than the relationship between the aims of people and their ability to achieve them.[141]

In general, people are more the product of their environment than of their genetic endowment. This environment is being rapidly distorted by industrialization. Mankind has so far shown an extraordinary capacity for adaptation. Man has survived with very high levels of sub-lethal breakdowns. Dubos[142] fears that

---

[140] ILTIS, Hugh, LOUCKS, Orie, ANDREWS, Peter. *Criteria for an optimum human environment*, in: Science and Public Affairs Bulletin of the Atomic Scientists, January, 1970, pp. 2–6. ENGEL, George L. *A unified concept of health and disease*, in: Perspectives in Biology and Medicine, Summer 1960, pp. 459–485.

[141] ANTONOVSKY, Aaron. *Breakdown: a needed fourth step in the conceptual armamentarium of modern medicine*, in: Social Science and Medicine, Vol. 6, 1972, pp. 537–544, calls for a fourth category in the conceptual tools of modern medicine, the recognition of breakdown. So far medicine has developed three major concepts for the control of diseases. First it was discovered that disease could be prevented by environmental public health measures, especially by exerting control on supplies of food and water. The second breakthrough came with the concept of immunization, preparing the individual for resistance. Both these approaches are based on the image of the dangerous agent. A third breakthrough came with the recognition of multiple causation; one succumbs to a given disease when a given agent interacts with a given host in a given environment: the task of medicine is to recognize and control these givens. According to Antonovsky even Dubos does not go explicitly beyond this concept of multiple causation, even though he stresses the need to enhance man's capacity to adapt to the stress threatening in specific diseases. Antonovsky suggests the ulterior concept of breakdown, and a definition which permits the operationalization of this global concept. For this purpose he proposes specifications for four facets which are common to all disease. 1. pain in disease might be absent, mild, moderate or severe; 2. handicap may be absent, distracting, moderate or severe; 3. it can be assessed in six ways relative to its acute-chronic character (no acute or chronic condition; mild chronic but not degenerative; acute but not life threatening; serious chronic but not degenerative; serious-chronic-degenerative; or acute and life threatening); and finally 4. it can be recognized by the medical profession in the place at which it occurs as requiring no help, watching or therapy. Thus 288 possible breakdown types have been established. For the author, 'a radically new question arises: what is the aetiology of breakdown? Is there some new constellation of factors which is a powerful predictor of breakdown?'

[142] DUBOS, René. *Man and his environment: biomedical knowledge and social action.* Pan American Health Organization. Scientific Publication No. 131, March 1966.

mankind will be able to adapt to the stresses of the second industrial revolution and over-population just as it survived famines, plagues and wars in the past. He speaks about this kind of survival with fear because adaptability, which is an asset for survival, is also a heavy handicap: the most common causes of disease are exacting adaptive demands. The health care system, without any concern for the feelings of people and for their health, simply concentrated on the engineering of systems that minimize breakdowns.

Two of the foreseeable and sinister consequences of a shift from patient-orientated towards milieu-orientated medicine are the loss of the sense of boundaries between distinct categories of deviance, and a new legitimacy for total treatment. Medical care, re-education, and psychic reconditioning are all different names for the human engineering needed to fit populations into engineering systems. As the health delivery system continually fails to meet the demands made upon it, conditions now classified as illness might soon develop into aspects of criminal deviance and asocial behaviour. The behavioural therapy used on convicts in the U.S.A. and the incarceration of political adversaries in mental hospitals of the U.S.S.R. indicate the direction in which the integration of therapeutic professions might lead: an increased blurring of boundaries between therapies administered with a medical, educational or other ideological rationale.

The time has come not only for public assessment of medicine but also for public disenchantment with those monsters generated by the dream of environmental engineering.[143] If contemporary medicine aims at making it unnecessary for people to feel or to heal, eco-medicine promises to meet their alienated desire for a plastic womb.

---

[143] For critical evaluation of ecologically oriented medicine, see: COCHRANE, note 13, MCLACHLAN, Gordon, MCKEOWN, Thomas, eds., note 3.

83

PART III
STRUCTURAL IATROGENESIS

5. THE DESTRUCTION OF MEDICAL CULTURES

MANKIND is the one living species whose members are aware of being frail, partly broken, and headed for total breakdown, i.e. death. The clearer this consciousness the greater the need for dealing symbolically with the inevitable. The well-being of men and women increases with their ability to assume personal responsibility for pain, impairment, and on their attitude towards death. Culture and health are but two names for the programme by which a social group lives so as to perfect the ability of its members to cope with threats from the elements and from other people.

To be able thus to identify culture with a health programme, I follow and elaborate the ideas of Clifford Geertz.[144] In speaking about culture we must avoid the pitfalls of the anthropological evolutionists who look for man with a capital M behind all the specifics of individual customs just as much as we must avoid those of the cultural relativists who dissolve man into each given culture. Man, unmodified by a particular place and companionship, simply does not exist. He has never existed in this skinned condition, nor could he, by the very nature of the case, ever survive in this way.[145] But to understand in what sense culture is

[144] GEERTZ, Clifford. *The impact of the concept of culture on the concept of man*, in: COHEN, Yehudi A., ed. Man in adaptation: the cultural present. Chicago, Aldine, 1968.

[145] Bibliographic orientation to the study of medical cultures: DUNN, F. L. *Traditional Asian medicine and cosmopolitan medicine as adaptive systems.* Mimeo 14 p. DUNN indicates an important bias in most published research on medical cultures. He claims that 95% of the ethnographic (and also anthropological) literature on health-enhancing behaviour and on the beliefs underlying it deals with curing and not with the maintenance and expansion of health. ACKERKNECHT, Erwin, H. *Natural diseases and rational treatment in primitive medicine,* in Bulletin of the History of Medicine, Vol. XIX, No. 5, May 1946, pp. 467–497, provides a dated, but still excellent, review of the literature on the functions of medical cultures. He provides convergent evidence that medicine plays a social role and has a holistic and unitarian character in primitive cultures that modern medicine cannot provide. POLGAR, Steven. *Health and human behaviour: areas of interest common to the social and medical sciences* in: Current Anthropology, 3 (2), April, 1962, pp. 159–205, gives a critical evaluation of each item, and the responses of a large number of colleagues

a necessary 'cocoon' for the coping ability of man, we must go beyond its products and focus on its function. Culture in this sense is best seen not as a complex of concrete behaviour patterns such as customs, usages, traditions, or habit clusters, but as a set of control mechanisms: plans, recipes, rules, and instructions, all of which govern behaviour. Man is the animal who has lost his instinct and is desperately dependent upon such extra-genetic, outside-the-skin control mechanisms without which human behaviour would be ungovernable and human balance un-

to his evaluation. See also POLGAR, Steven. *Health*, in International Encyclopedia of the Social Sciences, Vol. 6, pp. 330–336. Medical culture seen with the blinkers of the behavioural technician. PEARSALL, Marion. *Medical behavioral science: a selected bibliography of cultural anthropology, social psychology and sociology in medicine.* University of Kentucky Press, 1963. 134 p. SELIGMANN, S. *Die magischen Heil and Schutzmittel aus der unbelebten Natur mit besonderer Berücksichtigung der Mittel gagen den bösen Blick. Eine Geschichte des Amulettenwesens.* Stuttgart, Strecker und Schroeder, 2 Vols., 1922, and SELIGMANN, S. *Der böse Blick und Verwandtes. Ein Beitrag zur Geschichte des Aberglaubens aller Zeiten und Völker.* Berlin, 1910, 2 Vols. SELIGMANN's works are treasure troves. See also JAYNE, Walter Addison. *The healing gods of ancient civilizations.* N.Y., University Books, 1962. GRABNER, Elfriede. *Volksmedizin. Probleme und Forschungs-geschichte.* Darmstadt, Wiss. Buchg., 1974, provides an anthology of critical studies on the history of ethno-medicine. JAKOBOVITS, Immanuel. *Jewish medical ethics. A comparative and historical study of the Jewish religious attitude to medicine and its practice.* N.Y., Bloch Pub. Co., 1959. Third ed., 1967. PREUSS, Dr. Julius. *Biblisch-talmudische Medizin. Beitrag zur Geschichte der Heilkunde und der Kultur überhaupt.* 3 Aufl. Berlin, 1923. 735 p. ULLMANN, Manfred. *Die Medizin im Islam.* Leiden, E. J. Brill, 1970. LECLERC, Lucien. *Histoire de la médecine Arabe. Exposé complet des traductions du Grec. Les sciences en Orient, leur transmission à l'Occident par les traductions latines.* 2 vols. N.Y., Burt Franklin, 1971 (original, 1876). Preuss, Ullmann and Leclerc are introductions to semitic medicine. For ethno-medicine in South America see: ACKERKNECHT, Erwin H. *Medical Practices*, in: STEWARD, Julian Haynes. *Handbook of South American Indians. Vol. 5: The comparative ethnology of South American Indians.* U.S. Bureau of American Ethnology. Bull. 143, pp. 625–643. For North American aborigines see pp. 339–342 in: MILLER, Genevieve. ed. *Bibliography of the history of medicine of the United States and Canada, 1939–1960.* Baltimore, Johns Hopkins Press, 1964. POYNTER, F. N. L. *Medicine and culture.* Proceedings of a historical symposium organized jointly by the Wellcome Institute of the History of Medicine, London, and the Wenner-Gren Foundations for Anthropological Research, N.Y. London, Wellcome Inst., 1969. See Poynter for the conflict between metropolitan medicine and various traditions on all continents. For the same conflict in Latin America see: RUBEL, Arthur. *The role of social science research on recent health programmes in Latin America*, in: Latin American Research Review, Vol. 2. 1966, pp. 37–56, ZSCHOCK, Dieber. *Health planning in Latin America: review and evaluation*, in: Latin American Research Review, Vol. 5, 1970, pp. 35–56. The best guide into a medical library is BLAKE, John B., ROOS, Charles, ed. *Medical reference works 1679–1966*, a selected bibliography. Chicago, Medical Library Association, 1967.

attainable. Culture, in other words, is the particular form that survival, coping, and viability take in a given human group; which really means that it is identical with the Gestalt of the group's health. Rather than something added to a virtually finished human animal, it is one of the central ingredients in the production of the animal itself. In submitting themselves to governance by symbolically mediated programmes that determine the artefacts to be produced, the way social life is to be organized and expressed in categories and emotions, men and women determine, however unwittingly, the culminating stage of their biological destiny. In determining their health, they create their physical being, just as, more generally, by determining their culture, they create themselves.

In his explanation of culture as a programme, Geertz points out that both enlightened and classical anthropology miss the point. Each endeavours to construct an image of man as a model, an archetype, a Platonic ideal, or an Aristotelian form. Whereas enlightenment anthropology strips away the trappings of culture to find 'natural man', classical anthropology factors out the commonalities of culture and sees what is left as 'consensual man'; together they provide the basis for the current vision of health as normality and of sickness as deviance from a theoretical norm. Both transform individual eccentricity and distinctiveness into deviation, impairment, and sickness by insisting on the underlying, unchanging normative type of man as the formal object of scientific enquiry. The fundamental distinction between animal and human health is alien to both of these models.

To become human, the individuals of our species always needed to discover a particular programme by which to conduct themselves in their struggle with nature and neighbour. In this struggle they would often be on their own, but the weapons and the rules and the style for the struggle were supplied by the culture in which they grew up. Each culture evolved and defined the way of being human or healthy in its unique way. Each group's code suits a given genetic make-up, a given history, a given geography, and the necessity of facing a given set of other cultures. Each group's code changes according to this total environment. Along with the culture, men evolved, each learning to keep alive in this common cocoon.[146] Each culture not only provides instructions for tilling and fighting, but also a set of rules with which the individual could come to terms with pain, impairment, and death. How to interpret these three most intimate and basic threats and how to relate to others faced by them was an essential part of each viable culture. Man's sense of his own body is a gift of his culture.[147]

Modern cosmopolitan medical civilization denies the need for man's acceptance of pain, sickness and death. Medical civilization is planned and organized to kill pain, to eliminate sickness, and to struggle against death. These are new goals, and goals which have never before been guidelines for social life. From being essential experiences with which each of us has to come to terms, pain, sickness and death are transformed by medical civilization into accidents for which people must seek medical treatment. The goals of medical civilization are thus antithetical to every one of the cultures with which it is confronted when it is dumped, as part and parcel of industrial progress, on the so-called underdeveloped countries.

Traditional culture derives its hygienic function precisely from its ability to equip the individual to make pain tolerable, sickness understandable, and the life-long encounter with death meaningful. Most traditional health care was a programme for sleeping, eating, loving, working, playing, dreaming, singing and

[146] GEERTZ, see note 144. In Java people flatly say: 'To be human is to be Javanese.' Small children, boors, simpletons, the insane and the flagrantly immoral are said to be 'ndurung djawa' (not yet Javanese). A 'normal' adult capable of acting in terms of the highly elaborate system of etiquette, possessed of the delicate aesthetic perceptions associated with music, dance, drama and textile design, responsive to the subtle promptings of the divine residing in the stillness of each individual's inward-turning consciousness is 'ampun djawa' (already Javanese). To be human is not just to breathe, it is also to control one's breathing by yoga-like techniques so as to hear in inhalation and exhalation the literal voice of God pronouncing his own name, hu Allah.

[147] GREVERUS, Ina-Maria. Der territoriale Mensch. Ein literaturanthropologischer Versuch zum Heimatphänomen. Frankfurt am Main, Athenaum, 1972. MUHLMANN, W. E. Das Problem der Umwelt beim Menschen, in: Zeitschrift für Morphologia und Anthropologia, XLIV, 1952, pp. 153–181. GEHLEN, Arnold. Die Seele im technischen Zeitalter, Sozialpsychologische Probleme in der industriallen Gesellschaft. Hamburg, Rowohlt Taschenbuch, 1957. BERGER, P., BERGER, B., KELLER. The homeless mind. N.Y., Vintage Books 1974. PLUGE, Herbert. Der Mensch und sein Leib. Tübingen, Max Niemeyer Verlag, 1967. BUYTENDIJK, Frederik, J. Mensch und Tier. Tübingen, Rohwolt. BUYTENDIJK, Frederick J. Prolegomena einer anthropologischen Physiologie. Salzburg, Otto Müller.

suffering.[148] Most healing was a traditional way of consoling, caring, comforting, accepting, tolerating, and also of rejecting the afflicted.[149] 'Culture' and 'health programmes' can be distinguished only by those social scientists who identify 'medical culture' with sick care; they are concerned mostly with purging, bone-setting, exorcisms, tooth-pulling, trepanning, and birth, and they count this latter as sick care only because their own wives feel sick when they are with child. In fact, this aspect of culture, to which most academic research is dedicated, constitutes but a tiny fraction of its health-granting wholeness. Culture was the framework for habits which could become conscious in the personal practice of the virtue of hygeia; medical civilization is the code by which we submit to the instructions emanating from the therapist.

As the medical institution assumes the management of suffering, my responsibility for *my* and *your* suffering declines.[150]

[148] GUBSER, A. W. *Ist der Mittagsschlaf schädlich?* in: Schweizerische Medizinische Wochenschrift, Vol. 97, Nr. 7, 1967, pp. 213–216. WISWE, Hans. *Kulturgeschichte der Kochkunst.* Kochbücher und Rezepte aus zwei Jahrtausenden und einem, lexikalischen Anhang zur Fachsprache von Eva HEPP. München, 1970. VAN GULIK, Robert. *La vie sexuelle dans la Chine ancienne.* Paris, Gallimard, 1971. GARDINER, Edward M. *Athletics of the ancient world.* Oxford Univ. Press, 1930. MICHLER, M. *Das Problem der westgriechischen Heilkunde,* in: Sudhoff Archiv, 46, 1962. SIGERIST, Henry E. *Disease and music,* in: Civilization and disease. Univ. of Chicago Press, 1943, Chap. XI, p. 212 ff.

[149] SIGERIST, Henry E. *A history of medicine. I. Primitive and archaic medicine.* N.Y. Oxford Univ. Press, 1967. ACKERKNECHT, E. H. *Primitive medicine and culture pattern.* in: Bulletin Hist. Medicine, 1942, Vol. 12, pp. 545–74. Sigerist states that: 'Culture, whether or not primitive, always has a certain configuration ... The medicine of a primitive tribe fits into that pattern. It is one expression of it, and cannot be fully understood if it is studied separately.' Ackerknecht exemplifies this integration of culture and medicine in three tribes: the Cheyenne, Dobuan and Thonga. For a classical description of this integration see EVANS-PRITCHARD. *Witchcraft, oracles and magic among the Azandé,* London, Oxford Univ. Press, 1951. Part IV, 3.

[150] I here argue that health and my ability to remain responsible for my behaviour in suffering correlate. Relief of this responsibility correlates with a decline in health. SCHUTZ, Alfred. *Some equivocations in the notion of responsibility,* in: Collected papers, II, Studies in social theory, The Hague, Nijhof, 1964, pp. 274–276, suggests an important distinction with regard to the notion of 'responsibility': a man is responsible *for* what he did; on the other hand he is responsible *to* someone, that is the person or group or authority who makes him responsible, or answerable. Only if I feel subjectively responsible for what I did or omitted to do without being held responsible (answerable) to another person, will the consequences be not reprehension, criticism, censure or other forms of punishment inflicted on me by someone else, but regret, remorse or repentance. In theological terms, contrition and not attrition will be the result. The consequent states of grief, anguish, or distress

Culturally regulated, autonomous health behaviour is restricted, crippled, and paralysed by the expansion of corporate medical care. The effectiveness of persons and of primary groups in self-care is overwhelmed by the competing industrial production of a substitute value. The institutional balance between two modes of complementary production is disturbed, and will eventually be broken, by self-reinforcing corporate domination.

The increasing attachment and allegiance to therapy also affects the social character of a people. An idolatrous demand for manipulation comes to be identified with health care and replaces autonomous confidence in biological vigour, the wisdom of traditional rules, and the compassion of neighbours.[151] When dependence on the professional management of pain, sickness and death grows beyond a certain point, the healing power in sickness, patience in suffering and fortitude in the face of death must decline. These three regressions are symptoms of third-level iatrogenesis: their combined outcome is Medical Nemesis. In the next three chapters I will deal successively with the historical appearance of each of these symptoms.

---

are marks of the true sense of guilt which is phenomenologically something entirely different from the guilt feeling in psychoanalytic terminology. This distinction made by Schutz is fundamental if we are to avoid confusion in traditional everyday reality. It also permits us to underscore a way in which the ethics of 'industrialized' social reality are new. In an industrialized social reality, both my survival and the goals of my group depend on the malignant functioning of tools, institutions and instrumentalities which ultimately wreak total destruction on those in whose service they are employed. The individual is bound in responsibility *to* his group *for* the functioning of those destructive instrumentalities. An inextricable web of guilt and grief overwhelms the ethical categories of tradition. Alone this experience can barely be borne, and in the current political context it cannot be shared with the members of an action group. The only adequate response is often renunciation of benefits and at the same time exile from the group.

[151] The dependence of the patient on the anonymous institution manifests in the most painful way the structure which the class-conflict assumes at the present stage of industrial development. This has been argued by M. Foucault. See ex. gr.: FOUCAULT, Michel, et LES MEMBRES DU G.I.S. (Groupe Information Santé). *Medecine et lutte des classes*, in: La Nef, Vers une antimédecine? Paris, Tallandier, No. 49, 29th year, October-December 1972, pp. 67–73.

6 THE KILLING OF PAIN

WHEN the cosmopolitan medical civilization colonizes any traditional culture, it transforms the experience of pain. Medical civilization tends to turn pain into a technical problem and thereby to deprive suffering of its inherent personal meaning. People unlearn to accept suffering as an inevitable part of their conscious coping with reality and come to interpret every ache as an indicator of their need for the intervention of applied science. Culture confronts pain, deviance and death by interpreting them; medical civilization turns them into problems which can be solved by their removal. Cultures are systems of meanings, cosmopolitan civilization a system of techniques. Culture makes pain tolerable by integrating it into a meaningful system, cosmopolitan civilization detaches pain from any subjective or intersubjective context in order to annihilate it.[152]

A myriad of different virtues express the different aspects of fortitude that traditionally enabled people to recognize painful sensations as a challenge and to shape their own experience accordingly. Patience, forbearance, courage, resignation, self-control, perseverance and meekness each express a different colouring of the responses with which pain sensations were accepted, transformed into the experience of suffering, and endured. Duty, love, fascination, routines, prayer and compassion were just some of the means that enabled pain to be borne with dignity. Traditional cultures made everyone responsible for his or her own performance under the impact of bodily harm or grief. Pain was recognized as an inevitable part of the subjective reality of one's own body in which everyone constantly finds himself, and which is constantly being shaped by his conscious reactions to it. Suffering meant an autonomous performance under the impact of painful or anguishing sensations. People knew that they had to deal on their own with their migraine,

152 Formulation by FRIEDMANN F. in a letter to Ivan Illich, Munich, 26 June, 1974.

phantom limb or neuralgia. Culture determined their competence to live with their own recollection of past injuries and their certainty of unending vulnerability.[153]

This rich texture of patterned responses to present evil and universal threat is now being homogenized into a demand for the technical management of sensation, experience and expectations. Pain had formerly given rise to a cultural programme whereby individuals could deal with reality in those situations in which reality was experienced as inimical to the unfolding of their lives. Pain is now being turned into a political issue which gives rise to a snowballing demand on the part of anaesthesia consumers for artificially induced insensibility, unawareness, and even unconsciousness.

As long as pain was primarily an experience that had to be faced and suffered, its political function was to set limits to man-made abuses of man by man when these became intolerable. Now an increasing portion of all pain is man-made, a side-effect of strategies for industrial expansion. Pain has ceased to be conceived as a 'natural' or 'metaphysical' evil. It is a social curse, and to stop the 'masses' from cursing society when they are pain-stricken, the industrial system responds by delivering them medical pain-killers. Pain thus turns into a demand for more drugs, hospitals, medical services and other outputs of corporate, impersonal care and into political support for further corporate growth no matter what its human, social or economic cost.

In one way or another all cultures teach suffering as an art enabling one to deal in deep loneliness with the kind of physical pain that cannot be avoided. Medical civilization teaches that suffering is unnecessary, because pain can be technically elimi-

---

[153] The expression of physical pain as given in the arts is one means of reconstructing the pain-experience of past epochs. BRAUER, Ernest Hannes. *Studien zur Darstellung des Schmerzes in der antiken bildenden Kunst Griechenlands und Italiens.* Breslau, Diss. Univ. Halle, 1934. GARNAUD, F. *La douleur dans l'art,* in: Aesculape, 1957, p. 40 ff. SHERER, Wilhelm. *Der Ausdruck des Schmerzes und der Freude in den mittelhochdeutschen Dichtungen der Blütezeit.* Diss. Strassburg, 1908. 75 S. ALBERT, Christine Ottilie H. *Leiderfahrung ünd Leidüberwindung in der deutschen Lyrik des 17. Jahrhunderts.* Diss. Munchen, 1956.

[154] I quote from the introduction to POYNTER, F. N. L. editor, *Medicine and culture.* London, Wellcome Institute of the History of Medicine, 1969, pp. 2–3, 'For many centuries, reinforced by religious teaching and beliefs, the Christian West accepted suffering as a necessary part of spiritual discipline; now it is universally rejected. The state organization of medical care represents this rejection in a formal

nated.[154] I will show that this technical management of suffering must give rise to a new kind of horror.

The subject is better understood when the social situation in which pain occurs is included in the explanation of pain.[155] The experience of pain that results from pain messages received by the brain depends in its quality and in its quantity on at least four factors besides the nature and intensity of the stimulus, namely culture, anxiety, attention and interpretation. All these are shaped by social determinants, ideology, economic structure and social character. Culture decrees whether the mother or the father, or both, must groan when the child is born.[156] Circumstances and habits determine the anxiety level of the sufferer and the attention he gives to his bodily sensations.[157] Training and conviction determine the meaning given to bodily sensations and influence the degree to which pain is experienced.[158] It is well known that soldiers on the battlefield who consider their mutilation a relatively happy ending of their own battle careers reject morphine injections which they would consider absolutely necessary to allay their anxieties if a mutilation similar to their wound were inflicted on them in an operating room.

structure. . . . Has scientific rationalism removed the support of traditional customs and beliefs before anything was prepared to take their place? What has happened to other societies which encouraged hedonism for the semi-literate masses, and scepticism for all?' I doubt that such a precedent exists.

[155] SZASZ, Thomas S. *Pain and pleasure.* New York, Basic Books, 1957. (London, Tavistock, 1957.)

[156] DICK-READ, Grantly. *Childbirth without fear* Dell Paperback, 1962, (orig., 1944) deals with the impact of culture on the level of fear and the relationship between fear and pain-experience.

[157] BEECHER, Henry K. *Measurement of subjective responses: quantitative effects of drugs.* New York, Oxford University Press, 1959. Opiates exert their principal action not on the pain impulse which is transmitted through the nervous system, but on the psychological overlay of pain. They lower the level of anxiety. Placebos can achieve the same effect in many people. Severe post-surgical pain can be relieved in about 35% of patients by giving them a sugar or saline tablet, instead of an analgesic. Since only 75% are relieved under such circumstances with large doses of morphine, the placebo-effect might account for 50% of drug effectiveness. See also: HILL, Harris et al. *Studies on anxiety associated with anticipation of pain: I. Effects of morphine,* in: Archives of Neurology and Psychiatry, 67, 1952, pp. 612–619.

[158] WEBER, Leonhard M. *Grenzfragen der Medizin und Moral,* in: Gott in Welt. Festgabe für Karl Rahner, Vol. II, 1964, pp. 693–723. BRENA, Steven. *Pain and religion: a psychophysiological study.* C. C. Thomas, 1972. CONVEGNI DEL CENTRO DI STUDI SULLA SPIRITUALITA MEDIEVALE. *Il dolore e la morte nella spiritualità, secoli XII-XIII,* OH 7–10. 1962. Todi, Acad. Tudealina, 1967.

As culture is medicalized, the social determinants of pain are distorted. Whereas culture recognizes pain as an intrinsic, intimate and incommunicable 'dis-value,' medical civilization focuses primarily on pain as a systemic reaction that can be verified, measured and regulated. Only pain perceived in this objectivized form constitutes a diagnosis that calls for specific treatment. This objectivization and quantification of pain goes so far that medical treatises speak of painful diseases, operations, or conditions even in cases where patients claim to be insensible to them. Pain calls for methods of control by the physician rather than an approach that might help the person in pain to take on responsibility for his experience.[159] The medical profession judges [160] which pains are authentic, which have a physical and which a psychic base, which are imagined and which are simulated. Society recognizes and endorses this professional judgement. Compassion turns into an obsolete virtue. The person in pain is left with less and less social context to give meaning to the experience overwhelming him.

The history of medical pain has not yet been written. A few learned monographs deal with the moments during the last 250 years in which the attitude of physicians towards pain has changed,[161] and some historical references can be found in papers dealing with contemporary attitudes towards pain.[162] The existential school of anthropological medicine has gathered valuable insights into the development of modern pain while tracing the change of bodily perception in a technological age.[163] The relationship between the medical institution and the anxiety

---

[159] For information on this subject consult: HARDY, James D. et. al. *Pain, sensations and reactions.* 1967. Repr. of 1952 ed. Hafner. WOLFF, Harold G., WOLFF, Stewart. *Pain.* 2nd. ed. American Lecture Physiology series. 1958. C. C. Thomas. CRUE, Benjamin L. Jr. *Pain and suffering. Selected aspects.* C. C. Thomas, 1970.

[160] SZASZ, Thomas S. *The psychology of persistent pain. A portrait of l'Homme Douloureux,* in: SOULAIRAC, CAHN, CHARPENTIER. *Pain.* 1968, pp. 93–113.

[161] TOELLNER, Richard. *Die Umbewertung des Schmerzes im 17, Jahrhundert in ihren Vorraussetzungen und Folgen,* in: Med. Historisches Journal, 6, 1971. SAUERBRUCH, Ferdinand, WENKE, Hans. *Wesen und Bedeutung des Schmerzes.* Berlin, Junker und Dünnhaupt, 1936. KEYS, Thomas. *History of surgical anesthesia.* Revised edition, New York, Dover, 1963.

[162] KEELE, Kenneth D. *Anatomies of pain.* Oxford, C. C. Thomas, 1957. BUDDENSIEG, H. *Leid und Schmerz als Schofermacht.* Heidelberg, 1956.

[163] BUYTENDIJK, Frederick Jacobus Johannes. *De la douleur.* Bibliothèque de Philosophie Contemporaine, P.U.F. 1951. GEBSATTEL, Victor E. von. *Imago hominis. Beiträge zu einer personalen Anthropologie.* 2. edit. Otto Muller, Salzburg.

suffered by its patients has been explored by psychiatrists[164] and occasionally by general physicians but the relationship of corporate medicine to bodily pain in its strong sense is still virgin territory for research. One of the difficulties a historian of pain will encounter is the profound transformation undergone by the relationship of pain to the other ills man can suffer. Pain has changed its position in relation to grief, guilt, sin, anguish, fear, hunger, impairment, and discomfort. What we call pain in a surgical or cancer ward is something for which former generations had no special name. It seems as if pain were now only that part of human suffering over which the medical profession can claim competence or control.

A primary obstacle to a history of bodily pain, therefore, is a matter of language. The technical matter which contemporary medicine designates by the term pain even today has no simple equivalent in ordinary speech. In most languages the term taken over by the doctors covers grief, sorrow, anguish, shame and guilt. The English 'pain' and the German 'Schmerz' are still relatively easy to use in such a way that a mostly, though not exclusively, physical meaning is conveyed. Most Indo-Germanic synonyms cover a wider range of meaning.[165] Bodily pain is designated by terms that also extend to 'hard work', 'toil', 'trial', 'torture', 'endurance', 'punishment', or more generally, 'affliction', and extend their meaning to 'illness', 'tiredness', 'hunger', 'mourning', 'injury', 'distress', 'sadness', 'trouble', 'confusion', and 'oppression'.

This litany is far from complete: it shows that language can distinguish many kinds of 'evils', all of which have a bodily reflection. In some languages bodily pain is outright 'evil'. If a French doctor asks a typical Frenchman where he has a 'douleur', he will point to the spot and say 'j'ai mal là'. On the other hand,

[164] REIK, Theodor. Lust und Leid im Witz: sechs psychoanalytische Studien. Internationaler Psychoanalytischer Verlag, Wien/Leipzig, 1929/1930.
[165] See BUCK, Carl Darling. A dictionary of selected synonyms in the principal Indo-European languages. A contribution to the history of ideas. Chicago/London, Univ. of Chicago Press, 1949, for the following four semantic fields: pain-suffering 16.31; grief-sorrow 16.32; emotion-feeling 16.12; passion 16:13. See also: FRENZEN, W. Klagebilder und Klagegebärden in der deutschen Dichtung des höfischen Mittelalters. Würzburg, Diss. Bonn, 1938, 85 S. ZAPPERT, Georg. Über den Ausdruck des geistigen Schmerzes im Mittelalter, in: Denkschriften d. K. Akad. d. Wiss. Wien Phil. hist. Kl. 5, 1854. pp. 73–136.

a Frenchman can say: 'je souffre dans toute ma chair,' and at the same time tell his doctor 'je na'i mal nulle part.' If the concept of bodily pain has undergone an evolution in medical usage, it cannot be grasped simply in the changing significance of any one term.

A second obstacle to any history of pain is its exceptional axiological and epistemological status. Bodily pain is an intrinsic dis-value about which a peculiar kind of certainty exists.[166] As an intrinsic dis-value it is distinct from all extrinsic or systemic dis-values. In other words, my compassion is not the same for someone who himself says that he suffers as it is for someone else who is said to suffer; and I hardly sympathize at all with a statement about undefined patients with migraines. The 'pain' of which a history needs to be written is the first, the intrinsic, personalized experience designated by the expression 'my pain'. Nobody will ever understand 'my pain' in the way I mean it, unless he suffers the same headache, which is impossible, because he is another person. In this sense 'pain' means a breakdown of the clear-cut distinction between organism and environment, between stimulus and response.[167] It does not mean a certain class of experience that allows you and me to compare our headaches, much less does it mean a certain physiological or medical entity, a clinical case with certain pathological signs. It is not 'pain in the sternocleidomastoid' which is perceived as a systematic dis-value for the medical scientist.[168]

About this exceptional kind of dis-value that is pain, there exists an exceptional kind of certainty. Just as 'my pain' belongs in a unique way only to me, so I am utterly alone with it. I cannot

[166] HARTMAN, Robert S. *The structure of value: foundations of scientific axiology.* Carbondale, Southern Illinois University Press, 1967, p. 255 ff.

[167] BAKAN, David. *Disease, pain and sacrifice. Toward a psychology of suffering* Chicago, Beacon Press, 1968, deals with pain as a breakdown of *telos* and *distality.* 'Pain, having no other locus but the conscious ego, is almost literally the price man pays for the possession of a conscious ego... unless there is an awake and conscious organism, there is nothing one can sensibly refer to as pain.'

[168] BEECHER, H. K. *The measurement of pain,* in: Pharmacological Reviews, 9, 1957, p. 59, reviews 687 references. He concludes that pain cannot be satisfactorily defined, except as every man defines it introspectively for himself. Other useful surveys of literature on pain: NOORDENBOS, W. *Pain: problems pertaining to the transmission of nerve impulses which give rise to pain.* New York, Elsevier Publishing Co., 1959, and: MERKSEY, H., SPEAR, F. G. *Pain: psychological and psychiatric aspects.* London, Bailliere, Tindall and Cox, 1967.

share it. I have no doubt about the reality of pain-experience, but I cannot really tell anybody what I experience. I surmise that others have 'their' pains, even though I cannot perceive what they mean when they tell me about them. I am certain about the existence of their pain, because I am certain of my compassion for them. And yet, the deeper my compassion, the deeper is my certitude about the other person's utter loneliness in relation to his experience. Indeed, I recognize the signs made by someone who is in pain, even when this experience is beyond my aid or real comprehension. This awareness of extreme loneliness is a peculiarity of the compassion we feel for bodily pain which sets this experience apart from any other experience, for instance from compassion for the anguished, sorrowful, aggrieved, alien or crippled. In an extreme way, bodily pain lacks the distance between cause and experience found in other forms of suffering.

Notwithstanding the inability to communicate bodily pain, perception of it in another is so fundamentally human that it cannot be put into parentheses.[169] The patient cannot conceive that his doctor is a being who is unaware of his pain, any more than the prisoner can conceive the same about his torturer. The certainty that we share the experience of pain is of a very special kind, greater than the certainty that we share humanity with others. There have been people who have treated their slaves as chattels but even they recognized that this chattel was able to *suffer* pain. Slaves are more than dogs, who can be hurt but cannot suffer. No slaveholder ever has been able to think of his slaves as beings devoid of the ability to inflict pain maliciously on the master, something a dog could never do. Wittgenstein has shown that our special, radical certainty about the existence of pain in other people can co-exist with an inextricable difficulty in explaining how this sharing of the unique can come about.

It is my thesis that bodily pain, experienced as an intrinsic, intimate and incommunicable dis-value, includes in our awareness the social situation in which those who suffer find themselves. The character of the society shapes to some degree the personality of those who suffer, and thus determines the way they experience their very own physical aches and hurts as concrete pain. In this

[169] WITTGENSTEIN, Ludwig. *Philosophical investigations.* Oxford, 1953, p. 89 ff.

sense, it should be possible to investigate the progressive transformation of the pain-experience that has accompanied the
medicalization of society. The act of suffering pain always has
a historical dimension.

When I suffer pain, I am aware that a question is being raised.
The history of pain can best be studied by focusing on that
question. No matter if the pain is my own experience or if I
see the gestures of another telling me that he is in pain, a
question-mark is written into this perception. Such a query is as
integral to physical pain as the loneliness. Pain is the sign for
something not answered; it refers to something open, something
that goes on to demand the next moment: What is wrong? How
much longer? Why must I/ought I/should I/can I/suffer? Why
does this kind of evil exist, and why does it strike me? Observers
who are blind to this referential aspect of pain would be left with
nothing but reflex or instinctive reactions. They would be studying a guinea-pig, not a human being. A physician, were he able
to erase this value-loaded question shining through a patient's
complaints, might recognize pain as the symptom of a specific
bodily disorder, but he would not have come close to the suffering
that drove the patient to seek help.

Unfortunately, the development of this capacity to objectify
pain is one of the results of a university education for physicians.
By his training the physician is often enabled to focus on
those aspects of a concrete person's bodily pain that are accessible
to management by an outsider: the peripheral nerve-stimulation,
the transmission, the reaction to the stimulus, or even the anxiety
level of the patient. Concern is limited to the management of the
systemic entity.

The way most experiments on pain are conducted point in this
direction. Animals are used to test the 'pain-killing' effects of
pharmacological or surgical interventions, and the observations
made on mice are then verified in people.[170] As long as people
are used as experimental subjects and examined under experimental conditions that are as much alike as those in which the
mice had been tested, the same pain-killers give more or less

[170] SOULAIRAC, A., CAHN, J., CHARPENTIER, J., editors. *Pain*. Proceedings of the
International Symposium organized by the Laboratory of Psychophysiology,
Faculté des Sciences, Paris, April 11–13, 1967, especially pp. 119–230.

comparable results. But, more often than not, the effects of these procedures are completely out of line with those that have been found valid in experimental situations when the same drug or operation is used on people who actually suffer. In other words, it is only when the ability to suffer, to assume pain, has been deadened, that pain-killing works as expected. When pain-killing on prescription displaces the sense of inevitable suffering moderated by free access to analgesics, people unlearn to deal with their pains. 'Throw out opium, which the Creator himself seems to prescribe, for we often see the scarlet poppy growing in the cornfields, as if it were foreseen that wherever there is hunger to be fed there must also be pain to be soothed; throw out a few specifics which our doctor's art did not discover; throw out wine, which is a food, and the vapours which produce the miracle of anaesthesia—and I firmly believe that if the whole *materia medica*, as now used, could be sunk to the bottom of the sea, it would be all the better for mankind—and all the worse for the fishes.'[171]

Living in a society which values anaesthesia, both doctors and their potential clients are re-trained to smother pain's intrinsic question mark. The question raised by intimately experienced pain is transformed into a vague anxiety that can be easily reduced by opiates. Patients are trained to perceive their own pain as a clinically objective condition that can be submitted to treatment. Pain escapes our grasp; we can even submit to it without being able to suffer. Lobotomized patients provide the extreme example of this expropriation of pain: they 'adjust at the level of domestic invalids or household pets'. The patient becomes 'a house cat, but a warm, friendly tabby, rather than a snarling, frightened Siamese'. The lobotomized person still perceives pain, but he has lost the capacity to suffer from it; the experience of pain is reduced to a discomfort with a clinical name.

In order for an experience of pain to constitute suffering in the full sense, it must fit into a cultural framework. Precisely because culture provides a mode of organizing this experience, it provides an important condition for health care: it allows individuals to deal with their own pain. The act of suffering is shaped by culture into a question which can be stated and shared. Culture

[171] HOLMES, Oliver Wendell. *Medical essays*, Boston, 1883, quoted by Rick CARLSON.

provides the vehicle for expressing pain: the sounds and gestures that communicate and relieve. It also supplies the grammar to understand the pain as a challenge to be borne with dignity: the need to behave in a certain fashion distracts attention from otherwise all-absorbing sensations. Finally, culture supplies the myth with which to interpret pain: as Kismet to the Muslim, as Karma to the Hindu, as a sanctifying backlash of sin to the Christian, to others vengeance, punishment, the evil eye, or simply a mystery.

A medicalized culture assigns a role not only to an ailing person, but also to the physician faced by the one who is in pain. Although provided with the rationale for a respectful recognition of impotence when faced with certain kinds of pain, the medical scientist will be unable to acknowledge the question pain raises in the one who suffers. Such a doctor devalues the patient's pains into a list of complaints that can be collected in a dossier, but which leaves him exempt from responding to the person in pain with compassion.

One source of European attitudes towards pain certainly lies in Ancient Greece. The Greeks did not even think about enjoying happiness without taking pain in their stride. Pain was the soul's experience of evolution. The human body was part of an irreparably impaired universe, and the sentient soul postulated by Aristotle was fully co-extensive with his body. In this scheme there was no need to distinguish between the sense and the experience of pain. The body had not yet been divorced from the soul, nor had sickness been divorced from pain. All words which indicated bodily pain were equally applicable to the suffering of the soul.

The pupils of Hippocrates[172] distinguished many kinds of disharmony, each of which caused its own kind of pain. Pain thus became a useful tool for diagnosis. It revealed to the physician which harmony the patient had to recover. Pain might disappear in the process of healing, but this was certainly not the primary object of the doctor's treatment. Anaesthesia, as opposed to the

[172] For an exhaustive study of the diagnostic value ascribed to pain in Hippocratic literature see: SOUQUES, A. *La douleur dans les livres hippocratiques. Diagnostics rétrospectifs*, in: Bull. Soc. Franc. Hist. Med. 1937, 31, pp. 209–204; 279–309; 1938, 32, pp. 178–186; 1939, 33, pp. 37–38; 131–144; 1940, 34, pp. 53–59; 78–93.

solace of prayer, wine or poppy, was surprisingly absent from medical practice and from popular expectations. Whereas the Chinese tried very early to treat sickness through the removal of pain, nothing of this sort was prominent in the classical West. In view of our Greek heritage, it would be a grave mistake to believe that resignation to pain is due exclusively to Jewish or Christian influences. Thirteen distinct Hebrew words were translated by a single Greek term for 'pain' when 200 Jews of the second century B.C. translated the Old Testament into Greek.[173] Whether or not pain for the Jew was considered an instrument of divine punishment, it was always a curse. No suggestion of pain as a desirable experience can be found in the Scriptures or the Talmud.[174] It is true that very specific organs were affected by pain, but those organs were conceived of also as seats of very specific emotions, and the category of modern medical pain is totally alien to the Hebrew text. In the New Testament, pain is considered to be intimately entwined with sin. While for the classical Greek pain had to accompany pleasure, for the Christian pain was a consequence of his commitment to joy.

The history of pain in European culture would have to trace more than these classical and Semitic roots to find the ideologies which supported personal acceptance of pain. For the neo-Platonic, pain was interpreted as the result of some deficiency in the celestial hierarchy. For the Manichaean, it was the result of positive malpractice on the part of an evil demiurge or creator. For the Christian it was the loss of original integrity produced by Adam's sin. But no matter how much each of these religions might anathematize the others, for all of them pain was the bitter taste of cosmic evil, whether it was considered the manifestation of nature's weakness, of a diabolical will, or of a well-deserved divine curse. This attitude towards pain is a unifying and distinctive characteristic of Mediterranean post-classical cultures up until well into the seventeenth century. As an alchemic doctor put it in the 16th century, pain is the 'bitter tincture added

[173] For a dense treatment of bodily pain and suffering in the Bible, see: KITTEL, Gerhard. *Theologisches Wörterbuch zum Neuen Testament*, Stuttgart, 1933. The following articles: BULTMANN, *lype*; STAHLIN, *asthenés*; MICHAELIS, *pascho*. OEPKE, *nosos*.

[174] JAKOBOVITZ, Immanuel. *Attitude to pain*, in: Jewish medical ethics. New York, Bloch Publ. Co. 1967, p. 103.

to the sparkling brew of the world's seed'. Each person was born with the call to learn to live in a vale of pain.

This common ideological element of otherwise opposing religions set the stage for the experience of pain. Men recognized that in their personal pain they became aware of the bitter taste of the world's reality. The neo-Platonist interpreted bitterness as a lack of perfection, the Cathar as disfigurement, the Christian as a wound for which he was held responsible. In dealing with the fullness of life, which found one of its major expressions in pain, people were able to stand up in heroic defiance, or stoically deny the need for alleviation; they could welcome the opportunity for purification, penance or sacrifice, and reluctantly tolerate the inevitable while seeking to relieve it. Opium and alcohol have always been used. One approach to pain was unthinkable, however; that of killing or suppressing pain itself.

Toellner mentions three reasons why the idea of pain-killing was alien to all European civilizations. First: Pain was man's experience of a marred universe, not a mechanical dysfunction in one of its sub-systems. The meaning of pain was cosmic and mythic, not individual and technical. Second: Pain was a sign of corruption in nature, and man himself a part of that whole. One could not be rejected without the other; pain could not be thought of as distinct from the ailment. The doctor could soften the pangs, but to eliminate pain would have meant to do away with the patient. Third: Pain was an experience of the soul, and this soul was present all over the body. Pain was a non-mediated experience of lack or of evil. There could be no source of pain distinct from pain itself.

The campaign against pain got under way only when body and soul were divorced by Descartes. He constructed an image of the body in terms of geometry, mechanics or watchmaking, a machine that could be repaired by an engineer. The body became an apparatus owned and managed by the soul, but from an almost infinite distance. The living body of experience (to which the French refer in speaking about 'la chair' and the Germans in 'der Leib') was reduced to a mechanism which the soul could inspect.

For Descartes pain became a signal with which the body reacts in self-defence to protect its mechanical integrity. These reactions to danger are transmitted to the soul, which recognizes them as painful. Pain was reduced to a useful learning device: it now taught the soul how to avoid further damage to the body. Leibnitz sums up this new perspective when he quotes with approval a sentence by Regis, who was in turn a pupil of Descartes: 'The great engineer of the universe has made man as perfectly as he could make him, and he could not have invented a better device for his maintenance than to provide him with a sense of pain.'[175] Leibnitz's comment on this sentence is instructive. He first says that in principle it would have been even better if positive rather than negative reinforcement had been used by God, inspiring pleasure each time a man turns away from the fire that could destroy him. However, he concludes that God could have succeeded with this strategy only by working miracles, and since, again as a matter of principle, God avoids miracles, 'pain is a necessary and brilliant device to ensure man's functioning'. Within two generations of Descartes's attempt at a scientific anthropology, pain had become useful. It had turned from being the experience of the precariousness of existence into an indicator of specific breakdowns.

By the end of the last century, pain had become a regulator of bodily functions subject to the laws of nature and without any need for a metaphysical explanation.[176] It had ceased to deserve any mystical respect and could be subjected to empirical study with the purpose of doing away with it. Barely a century and a half after pain was first recognized as a mere physiological safeguard, the first medicine labelled a 'pain-killer' was marketed in La Crosse, Wisconsin, in 1853.[177] A new sensibility had developed

[175] LEIBNITZ, Gottfried Wilhelm. *Essais de Théodicée sur la bonté de Dieu, la liberté de l'homme et l'origine du mal.* Paris, Garnier-Flammarion, 1969. No. 342.
[176] RICHET, Charles. *Douleur,* in: Dictionnaire de physiologie. Vol. V, pp. 173–193. Paris, Félix Alcan, 1902. In his five volume standard dictionary of physiology he analyses pain as a physiological and psychological fact without considering either the possibility of its treatment or its diagnostic significance. Ultimately he comes to the conclusion that pain is supremely useful (*souverainement utile*) because it makes us turn away from danger. Every abuse is immediately followed for our punishment by pain, which is clearly superior in intensity to the pleasure that abuse produced.
[177] MATHEWS, Mitford M. editor. *A dictionary of Americanisms on historical principles.* Univ. of Chicago Press, 1966, 'pain-killer. Any one of various medicines or remedies for abolishing or relieving pain. 1853 La Crosse Democrat 7 June 2/4 Ayer's Cherry Pectoral, Perry Davis' Pain Killer. 1886 Ebbutt Emigrant Life 119. We kept a bottle of "Pain-killer" in the house . . . for medicinal purposes.'

which was dissatisfied with the world not because it was dreary or sinful or lacking enlightenment or threatened by barbarians, but because it was full of suffering and pain. Progress in civilization became synonymous with the reduction of the sum total of suffering. From then on, politics was taken to be an activity not so much for maximizing happiness as for minimizing suffering.[178] The result is a tendency to see pain as essentially a passive happening inflicted on helpless victims because the tool box of the medical corporation is not used in their favour.

In this context it now seems rational to flee pain rather than to face it, even at the cost of giving up intense aliveness. It seems reasonable to eliminate pain, even at the cost of losing independence. It seems enlightened to deny legitimacy to all non-technical issues that pain raises, even if this means turning patients into pets. With rising levels of induced insensitivity to pain, the capacity to experience the simple joys and pleasures of life has equally declined. Increasingly stronger stimuli are needed to provide people in an anaesthetic society with any sense of being alive. Drugs, violence and horror remain the only stimuli that can still elicit an experience of self. Widespread pain-killing increases the demand for painful excitation.

This raised threshold of physiologically mediated experience, which is characteristic of a medicalized society, makes it extremely difficult today to recognize in the capacity for suffering a possible symptom of health. The reminder that suffering is a responsible activity is almost unbearable to consumers, for whom pleasure and dependence on industrial outputs coincide. By equating all personal participation in reactions to unavoidable pain with 'masochism', they justify their passive life-style. While rejecting the acceptance of suffering as a form of masochism, anaesthesia consumers tend to seek a sense of reality in ever stronger sensations. They tend to seek meaning for their lives and power over others by enduring undiagnosable pains and medically unrelievable suffering by aspiring to the hectic life of a business executive or by becoming addicted to horror movies, or by actually producing the experience of bodily pain.

In such a society, to offer an ideal consisting of the culturally

[178] MINOGUE, Kenneth. *The liberal mind*. Methuen, London, 1963.

ordered self-management of unavoidable pains and minimum recourse to sedatives, narcotics and anaesthetics *in extremis* will be misinterpreted as a sick desire for pain.

Ultimately, the management of pain might substitute a new kind of horror for suffering: the experience of the artificially painless. Lifton describes the impact of mass death on survivors by studying people who had been close to ground zero in Hiroshima.[179] He found that people moving amongst the injured and dying simply ceased to feel; they were in a state of emotional closure, without emotional response. He believed that after a while this closure merged with a depression which twenty years after the bomb still manifested itself in the guilt or shame of having survived without experiencing any pain at the time of the explosion. These people live in an interminable encounter with death which has spared them, and they suffer from a vast break-down of trust in the larger human matrix that supports each individual human life. They experienced their anaesthetized passage through this event as something just as monstrous as the death of the people around them: as a pain which is too dark and too overwhelming to admit the question-mark.[180]

What the bomb did in Hiroshima might guide us to an understanding of the cumulative effect of a society in which pain has been medically 'expropriated'. Pain loses its referential character if it is dulled, and generates a meaningless, questionless residual horror. The suffering for which traditional cultures have evolved endurance sometimes generated unbearable anguish, tortured imprecations, and maddening blasphemies; these were also self-

---

[179] LIFTON, Robert J. *Death in life-survivors of Hiroshima.* New York, Random House, 1969.

[180] DES PRES, Terence. *Survivors and the will to bear witness.* Article from forthcoming book *The survivor*, Oxford Univ. Press, 1974, in: Social Research, Vol. 40, Nr. 4, Winter 1973, pp. 668–690, gives a constructive critique of LIFTON, Robert, v.n. According to him, the survivors of concentration camps have the urge to render significant a nameless experience they have known: pain which is utterly senseless. According to Des Pres their message is deeply offensive because since the middle of the 19th century the suffering of others has become charged with moral status. Kierkegaard preached salvation through pain, Nietzsche celebrated the abyss, Marx the downtrodden and oppressed. The survivor excites envy of his suffering, and simultaneously testifies that pain can be valued only by the privileged few. I propose an alternative explanation: the survivor is shunned because he feels impelled to call attention to the increase of utterly meaningless pain which is borne, not suffered, in industrial society.

limiting. The new experience that has replaced dignified suffering is artificially prolonged, opaque, depersonalized maintenance. Increasingly pain-killing turns people into unfeeling spectators of their own decaying selves.

7. THE INVENTION AND ELIMINATION OF DISEASE

THE French Revolution gave birth to two great myths: one, that physicians could replace the clergy; the other, that with political change society would return to a state of original health. Sickness became a public affair. In the name of progress it has now ceased to be the concern of those who are ill.[181]

For several months in 1792, the National Assembly in Paris tried to decide how to replace those physicians who profited from care of the sick with a therapeutic bureaucracy designed to manage an evil destined to disappear with the advent of equality, freedom and fraternity. The new priesthood was to be financed by funds expropriated from the church. It was to guide the nation in a militant conversion to healthy living which would make medical sick-care less necessary. Each family would again be able to take care of its members, and each village to provide for the sick who were without relatives. A National Health Service would be in charge of health care and would supervise the enactment of dietary laws and of statutes compelling citizens to use their new freedoms for frugal living and wholesome pleasures. Medical officers would supervise the compliance of the citizenry and medical magistrates would preside over health tribunals to guard against charlatans and exploiters.

Even more radical were the proposals from a sub-committee for the Elimination of Beggary. In content and style they are similar to some Red Guard and Black Panther manifestos demanding that control over health be returned to the people. Primary care, it was asserted, belongs only to the neighbourhood. Public expenses for sick care are best used to supplement the income of the afflicted. If hospitals are needed, they should be specialized: for the aged, the incurable, the mad, or foundlings.

---

[181] In this chapter I am quoting freely from documents gathered in the masterly study: FOUCAULT, Michel. *Naissance de la clinique, une archéologie du regard médical.* Paris, P.U.F. 1972.

Sickness is a symptom of political corruption and will be eliminated when the government is cleaned up.

The identification of hospitals with pestholes was current and easy to explain.[182] They were charitable institutions for the custody of the destitute. Nobody went to a hospital to restore his health. The sick, mad, crippled, epileptic, incurable, foundlings and recent amputees of all ages and both sexes were jumbled together; amputations were performed in the corridors between the beds. They were given some food, chaplains and pious lay folk came to offer consolation, and doctors made charity visits. Remedies made up less than 3% of the meagre budget. More than half went for the hospital soup; the nuns could get along on a pittance. Like prisons, hospitals were considered a last resort: nobody thought of them as tools for administering therapy to improve the inmates.[183] Logically, the Montagnards went beyond the recommendations made by the Committee on Beggary. Some demanded the outright abolition of all hospitals, saying that they are 'inevitably places for the aggregation of the sick and breed misery while they stigmatize the patient. If a society continues to need hospitals, this is a sign that its revolution has failed.'

The influence of Rousseau vibrates in this desire to restore sickness to its 'natural state': to bring society back to 'wild sickness' which is self-limiting and can be borne with virtue and style and cared for in the homes of the poor, just as previously the sicknesses of the rich had been taken care of. Sickness becomes complex, untreatable and unbearable only when

[182] For the history of the hospital see: RISLEY, Mary. *House of healing. The story of the hospital.* Garden City, N.Y. Doubleday, 1961. IMBERT, Jean. *Les hôpitaux en France.* Paris Coll. 'Que sais-je?', P.U.F., 1958. STEUDLER, F. *Le système hospitalier. Evolution et transformation.* Paris, Centre d'Etudes des Mouvements Sociaux, 1973. Mimeo. FERRY-PIERRET, Janine, KARSENTY, Serge. *Pratiques médicales et système hospitalier.* Paris, CEREBE, January 1974. JETTER, Dieter. *Geschichte des Hospitals.* Wiesbaden, Steiner Verlag, 1966. Südhoff Archiv, Beihefte, Heft 5, is planned for several volumes, clear and complete, strongly architecturally oriented. BURDETT, Henry. *Hospitals and asylums of the world: their origin, history, construction, administration . . . and legislation.* 4 vols., London, 1893, a monumental classic.

[183] For the history of betterment by incarceration consult: ROTHMAN, David. *The discovery of the asylum.* Boston, Little Brown and Co., 1971. KOTLER, Milton. *Neighborhood government: the local foundations of political life.* New York, Bobbs-Merrill Co., 1969 makes a clear case for Boston. See also: CARLSON, Rick J. *There are no cures in cages.* The Center Magazine, Santa Barbara, May–June 1974, pp. 27–31.

exploitation breaks up the family. It becomes malignant and demeaning with the advent of urbanization and civilization. The sickness seen in hospitals is man-made, like all forms of social injustice, and it thrives among the self-indulgent and those whom they have impoverished. 'In the hospital, sickness is totally corrupted; it turns into "prison fever" characterized by spasms, fever, indigestion, pale urine, depressed respiration, and ultimately leads to death: if not on the eighth or eleventh day, then on the thirteenth.' It is in this kind of language that medicine first became a political issue. The plans to engineer a society into health began with the call for a social reconstruction that would eliminate the ills of civilization. What Dubos has called the Mirage of Health began as a political programme.

In the public rhetoric of the 1790s, the idea of using bio-medical interventions on people or on their environment was totally absent. Only with the Restoration was the task of eliminating sickness turned over to the medical profession. After the Congress of Vienna, hospitals proliferated and medical schools boomed. So did the discovery of diseases. Illness was still primarily non-technical. In 1770, general practice knew of little besides the pest and the pox,[184] but by 1860 even the ordinary citizen recognized the medical name of a dozen diseases. The sudden emergence of the doctor as saviour, culture-hero and miracle worker was not due to the proven efficacy of new techniques but to the need for a magical ritual that would lend credibility to a pursuit at which a political revolution had failed. If 'sickness' and 'health' were to lay claim to public resources, then these concepts had to be made operational. Ailments had to be turned into objective diseases. Species had to be clinically defined and verified so that officials could fit them into wards, records, budgets and museums. The object of medical treatment as defined by a new, though submerged, political ideology acquired the status of an entity that existed quite separately from both doctor and patient.

We tend to forget how recently disease-entities were born. In the mid-19th century, a saying attributed to Hippocrates was still quoted with approval: 'You can discover no weight, no form

[184] MILLEPIERRES, François. *La vie quotidienne des médecins au temps de Molière.* Paris, Hachette, 1964.

nor calculation to which to refer your judgement of health and sickness. In the medical arts there exists no certainty except in the physicians' senses.' Sickness was still personal suffering in the mirror of the doctor's vision. The transformation of this medical portrait into a clinical entity represents an event in medicine that corresponds to the achievement of Copernicus in astronomy: man was catapulted and estranged from the centre of his universe.

Three centuries of preparation were required before this sudden emergence of disease could occur. The hope of bringing to medicine the perfection Copernicus had given astronomy dates from the time of Galileo. Descartes traced the co-ordinates for the implementation of the project. His description effectively turned the human body into a clockwork and placed a new distance, not only between soul and body, but also between the patient's complaint and the physician's eye. Within this mechanized framework, pain turned into a red light and sickness into mechanical trouble. A new kind of taxonomy of diseases became possible. As minerals and plants could be classified, so diseases could be isolated and put into their place by the doctor-taxonomist. The logical framework for a new purpose in medicine had been laid. Sickness was placed in the centre of the medical system, a sickness that could be subjected to (a) operational verification by measurement, (b) clinical study and experiment, and (c) evaluation according to engineering norms.

Galileo's contemporaries were the first to apply measurement to the sick.[185] They had little success. Since Galen had taught that urine was secreted directly from the vena cava, and that its composition was a direct indication of the nature of the blood, doctors had tasted and smelled urine and had assayed it by the light of both sun and moon. The 16th-century alchemists had learned to measure specific gravity with considerable precision, and they subjected the urine of the sick to their methods. Dozens

[185] For the history of measurements consult two symposia: WOOLF, Harry, editor. *Quantification: a history of the meaning of measurement in the natural and social sciences.* Bobbs Merrill, 1961, and LERNER, Daniel. *Quantity and quality. The Hayden Colloquium on scientific method and concept.* New York, Free Press of Glencoe, 1961. Particularly consult in WOOLF, Harry, the paper by: SHRYOCK, Richard H. *The history of quantification in medical science,* pp. 85–107. For the application of measurement to non-medical aspects of man, see: STEVENS, S. S. *Measurement and man,* in: Science, Vol. 127, No. 3295, 21 February, 1958, pp. 383–389, and STEVENS, S. S. *Handbook of experimental psychology.* New York, John Wiley & Sons.

of distinct and differing meanings were ascribed to changes in the specific gravity of urine. With this first measurement, doctors began to read diagnostic and curative meaning into any new measurement they learned to perform.

The use of physical measurements prepared for a belief in the real existence of diseases and their autonomy from the perception of doctor and patient. The use of statistics underpinned this belief. It showed that diseases were present in the environment, and could invade and infect people. The first clinical tests using statistics, which were performed in the U.S. in 1721 and published in London in 1722, provided hard data indicating that smallpox was threatening Massachusetts, and that people who had been inoculated were protected against its attacks. They were conducted by Dr. Cotton Mather, who is better known for his inquisitorial competence during the Salem witch trials than for this spirited defence of smallpox inoculation.

During the 17th and 18th centuries, doctors who applied measurements to sick people were liable to be considered quacks by their colleagues. During the French Revolution, English doctors still looked askance at clinical thermometry. Together with the routine taking of the pulse, it became accepted clinical practice only around 1845, thirty years after the stethoscope was first used by Laennec.

As the doctor's interest shifted from the sick to sickness, the hospital became a museum of sickness. The wards were full of indigent people who offered their bodies as spectacles to any physican willing to treat them.[186] The realization that the hospital was the logical place to study and compare 'cases' developed

---

[186] When disease became an entity which could be separated from man and dealt with by the doctor, other aspects of man suddenly became detachable, usable, salable. The sale of the shadow is a typically 19th century literary motif. (A. V. CHAMISSO. *Peter Schlemihls wundersame Geschichte*, 1814.) A demoniacal doctor can deprive man of his mirror image (E. T. A. HOFFMAN, 1815. *Die Geschichte vom verlorenen Spiegelbild* in: Die Abenteuer einer Sylvesternacht). In W. HAUFF (*Das steinerne Hertz* in Das Wirtshaus im Spessat, 1828) the hero exchanges his heart for one of stone in order to save himself from bankruptcy. Within the next two generations, literary treatment is given to the sale of appetite, name, youth and memories. See: FRENZEL, Elisabeth. *Schlemihl*, in: Stoffe der Weltliteratur. Stuttgart, Kroner Verlag, 1970, pp. 667–669. Note that this typical 19th century 'sale' is clearly distinct from the old Faust motif in which the soul after death belongs to the devil. DEDEYAN, Charles. *Le thème de Faust dans la littérature européenne*, 4 vols. Paris, 1954–1961.

towards the end of the 18th century. Doctors visited hospitals where all kinds of sick people were mingled, and trained themselves to pick out several 'cases' of the same disease. They developed 'bedside vision' or a clinical eye. During the first decades of the 19th century, the medical attitude towards hospitals went through a further development. Until then, new doctors had been trained mostly by lectures, demonstrations and disputations. Now the 'bedside' became the clinic, the place where future doctors were trained to see and recognize diseases. The clinical approach to sickness gave birth to a new language which spoke about diseases from the bedside, and to a hospital reorganized by disease for the exhibition of diseases to students.

The hospital, which at the very beginning of the 19th century had become a place for diagnosis, now turned into a place for teaching. Soon it would become a laboratory for experimenting with treatments, and towards the turn of the century a place for healing.[187] By now the pesthouse has been transformed into a compartmentalized repair shop.

All this happened in stages. During the 19th century, the clinic became the place where disease carriers were assembled, diseases were identified, and a census of diseases was kept. Medical perception of reality became hospital-based much earlier than medical practice. The specialized hospital demanded by the French Revolutionaries for the sake of the patient became a reality because doctors needed to classify sickness. During the entire 19th century, pathology remained overwhelmingly the classification of anatomical anomalies. Only towards the end of the century did the pupils of Claude Bernard also begin to label and catalogue the pathology of functions.[188] Along with sickness, health acquired a clinical status, becoming the absence of clinical symptoms. Clinical standards of normality became associated with well-being.[189]

[187] BERGHOFF, Emmanuel. *Entwicklungsgeschichte des Krankheitsbegriffes.* Wien, Maudrich, 1947.

[188] GRMEK, Mirko D. *La conception de la maladie et de la santé chez Claude Bernard,* in: KOYRÉ, Alexandre. *Mélanges Alexandre Koyré. L'aventure de la science,* Vol. 1, pp. 208–227. Paris, Hermann, 1964.

[189] CANGUILHEM, Georges. *Le normal et le pathologique.* Paris, P.U.F. 1972, is a thesis on the history of the idea of normalcy in nineteenth century pathology, finished in 1943 with a postscript in 1966. On the history of 'normality' in psychiatry see: FOUCAULT, Michel. *Histoire de la folie à l'âge classique.* Paris, Plon, 1961. English translation: *Madness and civilization,* New York, New American Library.

Disease could never have been associated with abnormality unless the value of universal standards had come to be recognized in one field after another over a period of 200 years. The value of such operationally fixed standards rose with the expansion of nation states. The first form of behaviour to be standardized was language. In 1635, at the behest of Cardinal Richelieu, the King of France formed an Academia of the forty supposedly most distinguished men of French letters for the purpose of protecting and perfecting the French language. In fact, they imposed the language of the rising bourgeoisie which was also gaining control over the expanding tools of production. The language of the new class of capitalist producers became normative for all classes. State authority had expanded beyond statute law to regulate means of expression. Citizens learned to recognize the normative power of an élite in areas left untouched by the canons of the church and the civil and penal codes of the state. Mistakes against the codified laws of French grammar now carried their own sanctions; they put the speaker in his place—that is, deprived him of privilege. Good French was that which rose to academic standards, as good health would soon be that which was up to the clinical norm.

'Norma' in Latin means square, the carpenter's square. Until the 1830s, the English word 'normal' meant standing at a right angle. During the 40s it came to designate things which were conforming to a common type. In the 80s in America it came to mean the usual state or condition, not only of things but also of people. Only in our century could it be used to evaluate people. However, in France the word was transposed from geometry into society a century earlier. 'École Normale' designated the school at which teachers for the Empire were trained. The word was first given a medical connotation around 1840 by Auguste Comte. He expressed his hope that once the laws relative to the normal state of the organism were known, it would be possible to engage in the study of comparative pathology.

During the last decade of the 19th century, norms and standards became fundamental criteria for diagnosis and therapy. For this to happen, it was not necessary that all abnormal features be considered pathological: it was sufficient that all pathological features be considered abnormal. Disease as deviance from a standard made medical intervention legitimate by providing an orientation for therapy.

The perception of disease as a deviance from the norm is now changing the doctor-hospital relationship for the third time.[190] I believe that we are in the midst of this transformation. Cotton Mather had first used statistics to describe the nature of disease. Medicine today uses them increasingly for diagnosis and therapy. The word 'clinic', which means bedside and has been expanded to mean the detached view taken by the doctor, now means a place where people come to find out if they ought or ought not to consider themselves sick. Society has become a clinic, and all citizens have become patients whose blood pressure is constantly being watched and regulated to 'within' normal limits.

The age of hospital medicine, which from rise to fall has not lasted more than a century and a half, is coming to an end.[191] The acute problems of manpower, money, access and control which beset hospitals everywhere can be interpreted as symptoms of a new crisis in the concept of disease. This is a true crisis because it admits of two opposing solutions, both of which make present hospitals obsolete. The first solution is a further sickening medicalization of health care, expanding still further the control of the medical profession over healthy people. The second is a critical, scientifically sound, de-medicalization of the concept of disease.

Medical epistemology is much more important for the healthy

---

[190] OFFICE OF HEALTH ECONOMICS. *Efficiency in the hospital service*. OHE publications, Studies on Current Health Problems, No. 22, 1967, London.

[191] For the history of medical ideas during the 19th century: LAIN ENTRALGO, P., *La medicina Hippocratica*. (Revista de Occidente), Alianza, 1970. LEIBRAND, Werner. *Heilkunde. Eine Problemgeschichte der Medizin*. Freiburg/Br., Alber Verlag, 1953. HARTMANN, F. *Der ärztliche Auftrag. Die Entwicklung der Idee des abendländischen Arzttums aus ihren weltanschaulich-anthropologischen Voraussetzungen bis zum Beginn der Neuzeit*. Göttingen, 1956. MERLEAU-PONTY. *L'oeil de l'esprit*, in: Les Temps Modernes, No. 184–185, Paris, 1961, p. 193 ff. MERLEAU-PONTY. *Phénoménologie de la perception*. Paris, 1945. LEIBRAND, Werner. *Spekulative Medizin der Romantik*. Hamburg, 1956. FREYER, Hans. *Der Arzt und die Gesellschaft*, in: Der Arzt und der Staat. Leipzig, 1929. FULOP-MILLER, René. *Kulturgeschichte der Heilkunde*. Bruckmann, Munich, 1937. ROTHSCHUH, K. E. Hrag. *Was ist Krankheit? Erscheinung, Erklärung, Sinngebung*. Wege der Forschung, Vol. CCCLXII. Darmstadt, Wissenschaftliche Buchgesellschaft. 18 historically important critical contributions of the 19th and 20th centuries to the epistemology of sickness, among them: C. W. HUFELAND, R. VIRCHOW, R. KOCH, F. ALEXANDER. TOELLNER R. will publish a parallel volume, *Erfahrung und Denken in der Medizin*.

solution of this crisis than either medical biology or medical technology. Such an epistemology will have to clarify the logical status and the social nature of diagnosis and therapy, primarily in physical—as opposed to mental—sickness. All disease is a socially created reality. What it means and the response it evokes have a history. The study of this history can enable us to understand the degree to which we are prisoners of the medical ideology in which we were brought up.

A number of authors have recently tried to debunk the status of mental deviance as a 'disease'. Paradoxically, they have rendered it more and not less difficult to raise the same kind of question about disease in general. Leifer, Goffman, Szasz, Laing, and others are all interested in the political genesis of mental illness and its use for political purposes.[192] In order to make their point, they all contrast 'unreal' mental with 'real' physical disease.

According to them, the language of natural science now applied to all conditions that are studied by physicians really fits physical sickness only. Physical sickness is confined to the body, and it lies in an anatomical, physiological and genetic context. The 'real' existence of these conditions can be confirmed by measurement and experiment. Such operational verification of 'real' sickness can be conducted—at least theoretically—without any reference to a value system. None of this applies to mental sickness: its status as a 'sickness' depends entirely on psychiatric judgement. The psychiatrist acts as the agent of a social, ethical and political milieu. Measurements and experiments on these 'mental' conditions can be conducted only within the framework of ideological co-ordinates, which derive their consistency from the general social prejudice of the psychiatrist. The prevalence of sickness is blamed on life in an alienated society, but while political reconstruction might eliminate much psychic sickness, it would merely provide better and more equitable technical treatment for those who are physically ill. This anti-psychiatric

[192] SZASZ, Thomas. *Myth of mental illness.* Harper and Row. 1961. SZASZ, Thomas. *Manufacture of madness: a comparative study of the inquisition and the mental health movement.* Harper and Row, 1970. LEIFER, Ronald. *In the name of mental health: social functions of psychiatry.* Science, 1969. GOFFMAN, Erving. *Asylums: essays on the social situation of mental patients and other inmates.* New York, Doubleday, 1973, (orig. 1961). LAING, R. D., ESTERSON, A. *Sanity, madness and the family.* Penguin, 1970.

stance, which legitimatizes the non-political status of physical disease by denying to mental deviance the character of disease, is a minority position in the West although it seems to be close to an official doctrine in modern China, where mental illness is perceived as political action. Maoist politicians are placed in charge of psychotic deviants. Bermann[193] reports that the Chinese object to the revisionist Russian practice of de-politicizing the political deviance of class enemies by locking them into hospitals and treating them as if they had a sickness which is analogous to an infection. They pretend that only the opposite approach can give results: the intensive political re-education of people who are now, perhaps unconsciously, class enemies. Their self-criticism will make them politically active and thus healthy. Here again, the insistence on the primarily non-clinical nature of mental deviance reinforces the belief that another kind of sickness is a material entity.[194]

Industrial society cannot function without providing its members with many opportunities to be diagnosed as suffering from real, substantive disease as a distinct entity. An over-industrialized society is sickening, in the sense that people do not fit into it. Indeed, people would rebel against it, unless doctors provided them with a diagnosis which explains their inability to cope as a health defect. Diagnosis transfers the reason for the individual's breakdown from the engineered environment to the organism which does not fit. Disease thus takes on its own substance within the 'body' of the person. The doctor shapes and defines it for the patient. The classification of diseases (nosology) that society adopts mirrors its institutional structure, and the sickness which is engendered by this structure is interpreted for the patient in the language the institutions have generated. The social origin of disease entities is the need industrialized people have to exonerate their institutions. The more treatment people

[193] BERMANN, Gregorio. *La santé mentale en Chine.* transl. from the Spanish by A. Barbaste. Paris, François Maspero, 1974. Original title: *La salud mental en China.* Ed. Jorge Alvarez, Buenos Aires, 1970.
[194] SEDGEWICK, Peter. *Illness, mental and otherwise. All illnesses express a social judgement,* in: Hastings Center Studies, Vol. 1, No. 3, 1973. pp. 19–40, points out that events constitute sickness and disease only after man labels them both as a deviance (conditions which are under social control). He promises to raise the episte-mological question about sickness in general in a book soon to be published by Harper and Row.

believe they need, the less can they rebel against industrial growth.

Until sickness came to be perceived as an organic or behavioural abnormality the patient could hope to find in the eyes of his doctor a reflection of his own anguish. What he now meets is the gaze of an accountant engaged in an input/output calculation.[195] His sickness is taken from him and turned into the raw material for an institutional enterprise. His condition is interpreted according to a set of abstract rules in a language he cannot understand. He is taught about alien entities which the doctor combats, but only just as much as the doctor considers necessary to gain the patient's co-operation in his engineering of interventions and of circumstances. Language is taken over by the doctors: the sick person is deprived of meaningful words for his anguish, which is further increased by linguistic mystification.

Iatrogenesis due to the doctor's control over the language of suffering is one of the major bulwarks of professional privilege. As soon as medical effectiveness is assessed in ordinary language, it immediately appears that most effective diagnosis and treatment does not go beyond the understanding that any layman can develop. The continued use of specialized language makes the deprofessionalization of medicine taboo.[196]

The overwhelming majority of diagnostic and therapeutic interventions which demonstrably do more good than harm have two characteristics: the material resources for them are extremely

[195] ISRAEL, Joachim. *Humanisierung oder Bürokratisierung der Medizin*, in: Neue Gesellschaft, 1974, pp. 397–404.

[196] For literature on the history of words used for health, healing, sickness and bodily dysfunctions see DORNSEIF, Franz. *Der deutsche Wortschatz nach Sachgruppen.* Berlin, De Gruyter & Co., 1970, sections 2.16–2.22 and 2.41–2.45. For the Indogermanic synonyms see BUCK, Carl D. *A dictionary of selected synonyms in the principal Indo-European languages.* Chicago and London, Univ. of Chicago Press, 1949, 3rd impression, 1971, sections 4.83–484. MOLL, Otto E. *Sprichwörter-Bibliographie.* Frankfurt Am Main, Vittorio Klostermann, 1958, lists 58 collections of proverbs in all languages dealing with 'health, sickness, medicine, hygiene, stupidity and laziness' pp. 534–537. STEUDEL, Johannes. *Die Sprache des Arztes. Ethymologie und Geschichte medizinischer Termini* is a history of medical language. GOLTZ, Dietlinde. *Krankheit und Sprache*, in: Sudhoffs Archiv 53, 3, 1969, pp. 225–269 compares the language of Babylonians, Greeks and German blue collar workers. The bureaucratic language used about sickness by doctors diverges increasingly from the ordinary language in which the sick formulate their complaints. See also BARGHEER. *Krankheit. Krankheitsnamen*, in: Handwörter des deutschen Aberglaubens, Vol. V, pp. 377–378.

cheap, and they can be packaged and designed for self-use or application by family members. The price of what is significantly health-furthering in Canadian medicine is so low that the money now squandered in India on modern medicine would suffice to make the same resources available in the entire sub-continent. On the other hand, the skills needed for the application of the most generally used diagnostic and therapeutic aids are so simple that the careful observation of instructions by people who personally care would probably guarantee more effective and responsible use than medical practice ever could. Most of what remains could probably be handled better by 'barefoot' non-professional amateurs with deep personal concern than by professional physicians, psychiatrists, dentists, midwives, physiotherapists or oculists.

When the evidence about the simplicity of effective modern medicine is discussed, medicalized people usually raise these objections: sick people are anxious and emotionally incompetent for rational self-medication: even doctors call a colleague to treat their sick child; and malevolent amateurs could quickly organize into monopoly custodians of scarce and precious medical knowledge. These objections are all valid if raised within a society in which consumer expectations shape attitudes to service, in which medical resources are carefully packaged for hospital use, and in which the mythology of medical efficiency prevails. They would hardly be valid in a world which aims at rationality.

A good recent example of the deprofessionalization of biological interventions is certainly provided by abortion. The pregnancy test represents the highest technology now packaged for self-application by laymen. The vacuum extraction method has rendered the interruption of pregnancies safe, cheap and simple. Recent technology has made legal prohibition of abortion as meaningless as are New England's puritan laws against masturbation. Laws which give doctors a monopoly on legal abortions are now as questionable as old church laws which tolerated adultery only when performed in brothels with certified prostitutes.

The deprofessionalization of medicine does not imply and the author should not be taken as advocating the disappearance of specialized healers. Nor should his thesis be read as denying genuine competence or opposing public scrutiny and exposure of malpractice. But it does imply a bias against the mystification of the public, against the mutual accreditation of self-appointed healers, against the public support of a medical guild and of its institutions, and against the legal discrimination by, and on behalf of, people whom individuals or communities choose and appoint as their healers. The deprofessionalization of medicine does not mean denial of public funds for curative purposes, but it does mean a bias against the disbursement of any such funds under the prescription and control of guild members. Deprofessionalization does not mean the abolition of modern medicine. It means that no professional shall have the power to lavish on any one of his patients a package of curative resources larger than that which any other could claim for his own. Finally, the deprofessionalization of medicine does not mean disregard for the special needs which people manifest at special moments in their lives: when they are born, break a leg, become crippled or face death. The refusal to license doctors does not mean that their services shall not be evaluated by the public, but rather that this evaluation can be done more effectively by informed clients than by their own peers. Refusal of direct funding to the more costly kinds of technical devices of medical magic does not mean that the state shall protect individual people against exploitation by ministers of medical cults; it means only that tax-funds shall not be used to establish any such rituals. Deprofessionalization of medicine means the unmasking of the myth according to which technical progress demands an increase in the specialization of labour, increasingly arcane manipulations, and increasing dependence of people on the right of access to impersonal institutions rather than on trust in each other.

8 DEATH AGAINST DEATH

IN every society the dominant image of death determines the prevalent concept of health.[197] Such an image, the culturally conditioned anticipation of a certain event at an uncertain date, is shaped by institutional structures, deep-seated myths, and the social character which predominates. A society's image of death reveals the level of independence of its people, their personal relatedness, self-reliance and aliveness.[198] Wherever the metropolitan medical civilization has penetrated, a novel image of death has been transplanted. Insofar as this image depends on the new techniques and their corresponding ethos, it is supra-national in character. But these very techniques are not culturally neutral;

[197] OLSON, Robert G. *Death*, in: Encyclopaedia of Philosophy, Vol. 2, 1967, pp. 307–309, New York, Macmillan, gives a short and lucid introduction to the knowledge of death and of the fear of death. FEIFEL, Herman, editor, *The meaning of death*, New York, McGraw Hill, 1959, gave a major impetus to the psychological research on death in the U.S.A. FULTON, Robert. *Death and identity*, New York, Wiley Inc., 1965, is an outstanding anthology of short contributions which together reflect the stage of English language research in 1965. LANDSBERG, Paul. *Essai sur l'expérience de la mort. suivi de problème moral de suicide*, Paris, Le Seuil, 1951, a classical analysis. ECHEVERRIA, José. *Réflexions métaphysiques sur la mort et le problème du sujet*. Paris, J. Vrin, 1957, a lucid attempt at a phenomenology of death. FERBER, Christian von. *Soziologische Aspekte des Todes. Ein Versuch über einige Beziehungen der Soziologie zur philosophischen Anthropologie*, in: Zeitschrift für Evangelische Ethnik, Vol. 7, 1963, pp. 338–360, a strong argument to render death again a serious public problem. The author believes that death repressed, rendered private, and a matter for professionals only, reinforces the exploitative class structure of society. A very important article. See also: JANKELEVITCH, Vladimir. *La mort*. Paris, Flammarion, 1966, and MORIN, Edgar. *L'homme et la mort*. Paris, Le Seuil, 1970.

[198] For the study of the antique death-image in our general context, the following are useful: GARRISON, Fielding H. *The Greek cult of the dead and the chthonian deities in ancient medicine*, in: Annals of Medical History, 1917, I, pp. 35–53. WALTON, Alice. *The cult of Asklepios*. Cornell Studies in Classical Philology, No. III, New York, Johnson Reprint Corp. 1965 (orig. 1894). BENZ, Ernst. *Das Todesproblem in der stoischen Philosophie*. Stuttgart, Kohlhammer, 1929. XI, Tübinger Beiträge zur Altertumswiss. 7. WACHTER, Ludwig. *Der Tod im alten Testament*. Stuttgart, Calwer Verlag, 1967. TOYNBEE, Jocelyn Mary Catherine. *Death and burial in the Roman world*. London, Thames and Hudson, 1971. SAUER, K. *Untersuchungen zur Darstellung des Todes in der griechisch-römischen Geschichtsschreibung*. Frankfurt, 1930. KROLL, J. *Tod und Teufel in der Antike*. Verhandlungen der Versammlung deutscher Philologen, 56, 1926. BLUMMER, Hugo. *Die Schilderung des Sterbens in der griechischen Dichtkunst*, in: Neue Jahrbücher des klassischen Altertums, 1917, pp. 499–512.

they assumed concrete shape within Western cultures and expressed a Western ethos. The white man's image of death has spread with medical civilization and has been a major force in cultural colonization.

The image of a 'natural death', a death which ought to come under medical care and find us in good health and old age, is a quite recent ideal.[199] In 500 years it has evolved through five distinct stages, and is now ready for a sixth mutation. Each stage has found its iconographic expression: (1) the 14th-century 'dance of the dead'; (2) the Renaissance dance at the bidding of the skeleton man, the so-called 'Dance of Death'; (3) the bedroom scene of the aging lecher under the *Ancien Régime*; (4) the 19th-century doctor in his struggle against the roaming phantoms of consumption and pestilence; (5) mid-20th-century doctors who step between the patient and his death; and (6) death under intensive hospital care. At each stage of its evolution the image of natural death has elicited a new set of responses that increasingly acquired a medical character. The history of natural death is the history of the medicalization of the struggle against death.[200]

[199] This chapter leans heavily on the masterful essays by Philippe Aries: ARIES, Philippe. *Le culte des morts à l'époque moderne,* in: Revue de l'Académie des Sciences morales et politiques, 1967, pp. 25–40. ARIES, Philippe. *La mort inversée. Le changement des attitudes devant la mort dans les sociétés occidentales,* in: Archives Européennes de Sociologie, VIII, 2, 1967. ARIES, Philippe. *La vie et la mort chez les français d'aujourd'hui,* in: Ethnopsychologie, 27 (1), March 1972, pp. 39–44. AEIES, Philippe. *La mort et le mourant dans notre civilisation,* in: Revue Française de Sociologie, XIV, 1, January-March, 1973. ARIES, Philippe. *Les techniques de la mort,* in: Histoire des populations françaises et de leurs attitudes devant la vie depuis le XVIIIe siecle. Paris, Le Seuil, 1971, pp. 373–398. A synopsis in English: ARIES, Philippe. *Western attitudes towards death: from the Middle Ages to the present.* A lecture at Johns Hopkins University. Translated by Patricia Ranum. Johns Hopkins University Press, 1974. *La mort inversée* appeared as *Death inside out* in Hastings Center Studies, May 1974, Vol. 2, No. 2, pp. 3–18 (the bibliography is absent from the translation).

[200] In this chapter I am interested, above all, in the image of 'natural death'. I am using the term 'natural death' because I find it widely used between the sixteenth and the early twentieth century. I oppose it to 'primitive death' which comes through the activities of some fey, eerie, supernatural or divine agent, and to 'contemporary death' which more often than not is conceived as the result of a social injustice, as the outcome of class-struggle or of imperial domination. I am interested in the *image* of this natural death, and its evolution during the four centuries in which it was common in Western civilizations. I owe the idea of approaching my subject in this way to Werner FUCHS, *Todesbilder in der modernen Gesellschaft.* Frankfurt am Main, Suhrkamp, 1969. On my disagreement with the author, see footnote 239.

The Devotional Dance of the Dead

From the 4th century onwards, the Church had been struggling against the pagan tradition of crowds dancing in cemeteries: naked, frenzied and brandishing swords. Nevertheless, the frequency of ecclesiastical prohibitions testify that they were of little avail, and for a thousand years Christian churches and cemeteries remained dance floors. Death was an occasion for the renewal of life. The dance with the dead over their tombs was an occasion for affirming the joy of being alive and a source of many erotic songs and poems.[201] By the late 14th century, the sense of these dances seems to have changed:[202] from an encounter between the living and those who were already dead, it was transformed into a meditative, introspective experience. In 1424 the first Dance of the Dead was painted on a cemetery wall in Paris. The original of the 'Cimetière des Innocents' is lost, but good copies allow us to reconstruct it: king, peasant, pope, scribe and maiden each dance with a corpse. Each partner is a mirror image of the other in dress and feature. In the shape of his body Everyman carries his own death with him and dances with it through his life. During the late Middle Ages, indwelling[203]

[201] OHM, Thomas. *Die Gebetsgebärden der Völker und das Christentum*. Leiden, Brill, 1948, p. 372 ff, especially pp. 389–390, collects evidence on dances held in cemeteries and the struggle of the church authorities against them. A medical history of occidental religious choreomania: BACKMAN, E. L. *Religious dances in the Christian church and in popular medicine*. Stockholm, 1948. English translation by E. Classen, London, Allen and Unwin, 1952. Bibliography of the religious aspects of dancing: BERTAUD, Emile. *Danse religieuse*, in: Dictionnaire de Spiritualité. Fasc. XVIII–XIX, pp. 21–37. SCHIMMEL, A. *Tanz. I. Religionsgeschichtlich*, in: Die Religion in Geschichte und Gegenwart. Tübingen, 1962. Vol. 6, pp. 612–614. For the history of dances in or around Christian churches see: GOUGAUD, L. *La danse dans les églises*, in: Revue d'Histoire Ecclésiastique, t. 15, 1914, pp. 5–22; 229–245. BALOCH, J. *Tänze in Kirche und Kirchhöfen*, in: Niederdeutsche Zeitschrift für Volkskunde, 1928. SPANKE, H. *Tanzmusik in der Kirche des Mittelalters*, in: Neuphilosophische Mitteilungen, 31, 1930. Germanic precedents to Christian cemetery dances: WOLFRAM, R. *Schwerttanz und Männerbund*. Kassel, 1937. (Only partly in print.) DANCKERT, Werner. *Totengräber*, in: *Unehrliche Leute. Die verfehmten Berufe*. Bern, Franck Verlag, 1963, pp. 50–56.

[202] HUIZINGA, Jan. *La vision de la mort*, in: Le déclin du moyen age. Paris, Payot, 1932. Chapter XI, pp. 164–180.

[203] LADNER, Gerhart B. *The idea of reform. Its impact on Christian thought and action in the age of the Fathers*. Harvard Univ. Press, 1959. Consult p. 163 for the two currents within the Church about the relation of death to nature since the fourth century. For Pelagius death was not a punishment for sin, and Adam would have died even had he not sinned. In this he differs from Augustine's doctrine that Adam

death faces man; each death comes with the symbol of rank corresponding to his victim: for the king a crown, for the peasant a pitchfork. After dancing with dead ancestors over their graves, people turned to representing a world in which everyone dances through life embracing his own mortality. Death was not represented as an anthropomorphic figure but as a macabre self-consciousness, a constant awareness of the gaping grave. It is not yet the skeleton man of the next century to whose music men and women will soon dance through the autumn of the Middle Ages, but rather each decaying one's own aging and rotting self.[204] At this time the mirror becomes important in everyday life, and in the grip of the 'mirror of death' life acquires an hallucinating poignancy. With Chaucer and Villon, death becomes as intimate and sensual as pleasure and pain.

Primitive societies conceived of death as the result of an intervention by an alien actor. They did not attribute personality to death. Death is the outcome of someone's evil intention. This somebody who causes death might be a neighbour who, in envy, looks at you with an evil eye, or it might be a witch, an ancestor who comes to pick you up, or the black cat that crossed your path.[205] Throughout the Christian and Islamic Middle Ages,

had been given immortality as a special gift from God, and even more from those Greek Church Fathers according to whom Adam had a spiritual, or 'resurrectional' body before he transgressed.

[204] So far the deceased had appeared ageless on his funeral monument. He now appears as a decaying corpse. TRICOT-ROYER. Les gisants macabres de Boussu, Bruxelles, Vilvorde, Strasbourg, Beanne, Troyes, Enkhuyzen, in: Bull. Soc. Franc. Hist. Med. Vol. 20, pp. 85-99; 199-205. HORNUNG, J. P. Ein Beitrag zur Ikonographie des Todes. Diss. Freiburg, 1902. The encounter between the living and the dead takes on importance in a new literary genre: GLIXELLI, Stefan. Les cinq poèmes des trois morts et des trois vifs. Paris, 1914. EGILSRUD, S. J. Le dialogue des morts dans les littératures francaise, allemande et anglaise. Paris, 1934. KAULFUSS-DIESCH. Totengespräche, in: Reallexikon der Deutschen Literaturgeschichte, 3, p. 379 ff. and finds a new visual expression: KUNSTLE, K. Die Legende der drei Lebenden und der drei Toten. 1908. ROTZLER, Willy. Die Begegnung der drei Lebenden und der drei Toten. Ein Beitrag zur Forschung über mittelalterliche Verganglichkeitsdarstellung. Wintertur, Keller, 1961. MICHAULT, Pierre. Pas de la mort. Ed. Jules Petit, Soc. des Bibliophiles de Belgique, 1869. FREYBE, Albert. Das memento mori in deutscher Sitte, bildlicher Darstellung und Volksglauben, deutsche Sprache, Dichtung und Seelsorge. Gotha 1909. The fact that around 1500 death assumes strong skeletal features and a new autonomy does not mean that it had not always borne anthropomorphic features, if not in art, then in legend and poetry. GEIGER, Paul. Tod. 4. Der Tod als Person, in: Handwörterbuch des deutschen Aberglaubens. Vol. VIII, pp. 976-985.

[205]For contemporary bibliography on attitudes towards death among primitive people see: HERZOG, Edgar. Psyche und Tod. Wandlungen des Todesbildes in Mythos

death continued to be regarded as the result of a deliberate personal intervention of God. No figure of 'a' death appears at the deathbed, only an angel and a devil struggling over the soul escaping from the dying woman's mouth. Only during the 15th century were the conditions ripe for a change in this image,[206] and for the appearance of what would later be called a 'natural death'. The dance of the dead represents this readiness. Death can now become an inevitable, intrinsic part of human life, rather than the decision of a foreign agent. Death becomes autonomous and for three centuries coexists as a separate agent with the immortal soul, divine providence, angels and demons.

The Danse Macabre

In the morality plays,[207] death appears in a new costume and role. By the end of the 15th century, no longer just a mirror image, he assumes the leading role among the 'last four things', preceding judgement, heaven and hell.[208] Nor is he any longer

---

und in den Träumen heutiger Menschen. Zurich, 1960. (English translation: *Psyche and death*. Putnam, 1967.) Death is always conceived of as the result of an intervention by an agent. For the purposes of my argument the nature of this agent is unimportant. Though dated, HERTZ, Robert. *Contribution à une étude sur la représentation collective de la mort*, in: L'Année Sociologique, 10, 1905/1906, pp. 48–137, remains the best repository for older literature on this point. Complement with: HARTLAND, LANGDON, DE LA VALLÉE POUSSIN., et al. *Death and disposal of the dead*, in: Encyclopaedia of Religion and Ethics, Vol. IV, pp. 411–511. MOSS, Rosalind. *The life after death in Oceania and the Malay Archipelago*. 1925. Reprod. University Microfilms, Ann Arbor, 1972, shows that the burial forms tend to influence beliefs about the cause of death and the nature of afterlife. KELSEN, Hans. *Seele und Recht*, in: Aufsätze zur Ideologiekritik. Neuwied am Rhein und Berlin, 1964, suggests that the universal fear of murderous ancestors underpins social control. Consult also: FRAZER, James George. *Man, God and immortality*. London, Macmillan, 1927. FRAZER, James George. *The belief in immortality and the worship of the dead*. Vol. 1: the belief among the aborigines of Australia, the Torres straits islands, New Guinea and Melanesia. London, Macmillan, 1913. FRAZER, James George. *Fear of the dead in primitive religion*, London, Macmillan, 1936. LEVI-STRAUSS, Claude. *La pensée sauvage*. Paris, Plon, 1962, especially pp. 44–46; 314–333. FREUD, Sigmund. *Totem und Tabu. Einige Übereinstimmungen im Seelenleben der Wilden und der Neurotiker*. Frankfurt am Main und Hamburg, 2. Edit. 1961.

[206] BOSSUAT, Robert. *Manuel bibliographique de la litérature française du moyen age. Danse macabre* Nos. 3577–3580; 7013.

[207] For the evolution of the Jederman motif see: LINDNER, H. *Hugo von Hoffmannstahls 'Jederman' und seine Vorgänger*. Diss. Leipzig, 1928.

[208] TENENTI, Alberto. *Il senso della morte e l'amore nella vita del Rinascimento*, Torino, Einaudi, 1957. TENENTI, Alberto. *La vie et la mort à travers l'art du XVe siècle*. Paris, Colia, 1962.

just one of the four apocalyptic riders from Romanesque reliefs, or the bat-like Maegera who picks up souls from the cemetery of Pisa, or a mere messenger executing the orders of God. Death has become an independent figure who calls each man, woman, and child, first as a messenger from God but soon insisting on his own sovereign rights. By 1538 Hans Holbein the Younger[209] had published the first picture book of death, which was to become a best-seller: woodcuts on the *Danse Macabre*.[210] The dance partners have shed their putrid flesh and turned into naked

[209] HOLBEIN, Hans the Younger. *The dance of death. A complete facsimile of the original 1538 edition of Les simulachres et histoires faces de la mort.* New York, Dover Publ., 1971.

[210] REHM, Walter, *Der Todesgedanke in der deutschen Dichtung vom Mittelalter bis zur Romantik,* Tübingen, Max Niemeyer Verlag, 1967, gives evidence of a major change in the image of death in literature around the year 1400 and then again around 1520. See also DUBRUCK, E. *The theme of death in French poetry of the middle ages and the Renaissance.* The Hague, 1964, and KURTZ, L. P. *The dance of death and the macabre spirit in European literature.* New York, 1934. For the new death image of the rising middle classes of the late Middle Ages see: HIRSCH, Erna. *Tod und Jenseits im Spätmittelalter. Zugleich ein Beitrag zur Kulturgeschichte des deutschen Bürgertums.* Berlin, 1927. XIII, Diss. Univ. Marburg. Specifically on the Dance of Death. ROSENFELD, Hellmut. *Der mittelalterliche Totentanz. Entstehung, Entwicklung, Bedeutung.* Münster Köln 1954, Bohlau Verlag. IX, illustrated. (Beihefte zum Archiv fur Kulturgeschichte H.3.) Besprechung bei Frederick P. Pickering. ROSENFELD, Hellmut. *Der Totentanz in Deutschland, Frankreich und Italien,* in: Littérature Moderne 5, 1954, pp. 62–80. Rosenfeld is the best introduction to the research and gives a detailed up-to-date bibliography. For older literature complement with MASSMAN, H. F. *Literatur der Totentänze. Beitrag zum Jubeljahr der Buchdruckerkunst. Aus dem Serapeum besonders abgedruckt.* Leipzig, T. O. Weipel, 1840. See also: BUCHHEIT, Gert. *Der Totentanz, seine Entstehung und Entwicklung.* Berlin, 1926. STAMMLER, Wolfgang. *Die Totentänze des Mittelalters.* München, 1922, and CLARK, James M. *The dance of death in the middle ages and the Renaissance.* 1950. KOSAKY's three volumes: KOSAKY, Stephen P. *Geschichte der Totentänze,* 1. Lieferung: Anfänge der Darstellungen des Vergänglichkeitsproblems, 2. Lieferung: Danse macabre (with 27 illustrations) Einleitung: Die Todesdidaktik der Vortotentanzzeit, 3. Lieferung: der Totentanz von heute, Budapest 1936, 1941, 1944, Bibliotheca Humanitatis Historica I, V, VII, contain a mine of information, quotations from ancient texts and nearly 700 pictures of the dance of death up to the Second World War. SAUGNIEUX, J. *L'iconographie de la mort chez les graveurs français du XVe siècle,* 1974, and SAUGNIEUX, J. *Danses macabres de France et d'Espagne et leurs prolongements litéraires.* Fasco. XXX, Bibl. de la Faculté des Lettres de Lyon. Paris, Les Belles Lettres, 1972. BRIESENMEISTER, Dietrich. *Bilder des Todes.* Unterscheidheim 1970. Verlag W. Elf. Reproductions are very clear, and organized according to different themes. WARTHIN, Alfred Scott. *The physician of the dance of death.* Five parts published in: Annals of Medical History, New series. Vol. II, No. 4, July 1930, pp. 351–371; Vol. II, No. 5, Sept., 1930, pp. 453–469; Vol. 2, No. 6, Nov., 1930. pp. 697–710. Vol. III, No. 1, January 1931, pp. 75–109; Vol. III, No. 2, March 1931, pp. 134–165, deals exclusively with the physician in the Dance of Death. BLOCK, Werner. *Der Arzt und der*

skeletons. The representation of each man entwined with his own mortality has turned into a frenzied exhaustion in the grip of a force of nature. The intimate mirror image coloured by the 'new devotion' of the German mystics has been replaced by an egalitarian force of nature, the executioner of a law that whirls everyone along and then mows them down. From a life-long encounter, death has turned into the event of a moment.

Death here becomes the point at which linear clock-time ends and eternity meets man, whereas during the Middle Ages eternity had been, together with God's presence, immanent in history. The world has ceased to be a sacrament of this presence; with Luther it became the place of corruption that God saves. The proliferation of clocks symbolizes this change in consciousness. With the predominance of serial time, concern for its exact measurement and the recognition of the simultaneity of events, a new framework for the recognition of personal identity is manufactured. The identity of the person is sought in reference to a sequence of events rather than in the completeness of one's life span. Death ceases to be the end of a whole and becomes an interruption in the sequence.[211]

Skeleton men predominate on the title pages of the first fifty

Tod in Bildern aus sechs Jahrhunderten, Stuttgart, Enke Verlag, 1966, studies the doctor's encounter with death, in and outside of a formal dance. Consult the standard iconographies on Western Christian art: KUNSTLE, Karl *Ikonographie der christlicher Kunst*. Freiburg, Herder, 1926–1928. 2 vols. and MALE, Emile. *L'art religieux à la fin du moyen-âge en France. Étude sur l'iconographie du moyen âge et sur ses sources d'inspiration*. Chapter II, p. 346, La mort (see also the three other volumes on religious art in France). Compare Eastern iconography (Mt. Athos): DIDRON, M. *Manuel d'iconographie chrétienne, grècque et latine* with an introduction and notes by M. Didron, translated from a Byzantine manuscript. 'Le guide de la peinture' by P. Durand, Paris, Imprimerie Royale, 1845. BOASE, T. S. R. *Death in the middle ages. Mortality, judgement and remembrance*. London, Thames and Hudson, 1972.

[211] See: PLESSNER. Helmuth. *On the relation of time to death*, in: CAMPBELL, J. editor, Man and time, 1951. Papers from the Eranos Yearbook, Bollingen series XXX, 3. Pantheon Books, 1957, pp. 233–263, especially p. 255. On the impact of time on the French death-image see: GLASSER, Richard. *Time in French life and thought*. Transl. by C. G. Pearson. Manchester Univ. Press, 1972, in particular p. 158 and chapter 3, 'The concept of time in the later middle ages' pp. 70–132. On the growing impact which time-consciousness had on the sense of finitude and death see: HAHN, Alois. *Einstellungen zum Tod und ihre soziale Bedingtheit. Eine soziologische Untersuchung*. Stuttgart, Enke Verlag, 1968, especially pp. 21–84. KEERLOO, Joost A. M. *The time sense in psychiatry*, in FRASER, J. T. editor. The voices of Time. New York, George Braziller, 1966, pp. 235–252, and pp. 242–252. GIEDION, Sigfried. *Space, time and architecture. The growth of a new tradition*, 4th. rev. ed. Harvard, 1962.

years of the woodcut, as naked women now predominate on magazine covers. Death holds the hour glass or strikes the tower clock.[212] Many a bell clapper was shaped like a bone. The new machine, which can make time of equal length, day and night, also puts all people under the same law. By the time of the Reformation, post-mortem survival has ceased to be a trans-figured continuation of life here below, and has become either a frightful punishment in the form of hell or a totally unmerited gift from God in heaven. Indwelling grace had been turned into justification by faith alone. Thus during the 16th century, death ceases to be conceived of primarily as a transition into the next world, and the accent is placed on the end of this life.[213] The open grave looms much larger than the doors of heaven or hell and the encounter with death has become more certain than immortality, more just than king, pope, or even God. Rather than life's aim, it has become the end of life.

The finality, immanence and intimacy of personal death was not only part of the new sense of time, but also of the emergence of a new sense of individuality. On the pilgrim's path from the Church Militant on earth to the Church Triumphant in heaven, death was experienced very much as an event that concerned both communities. Now each man faced his own and final death. Of course, once death had become such a natural force, people wanted to master it by learning the art or the skill of dying. *Ars Moriendi*, one of the first printed do-it-yourself manuals on the market, remained a best-seller in various versions for the next two hundred years. Many people learned to read by deciphering it. Solicitous to provide guidance for the 'complete gentleman', Caxton published the *Art and Craft to Knowe ye Well to Dye* in 1491 at the Westminster Press. Printed in neat Gothic type, it became exceedingly popular. Editions were made from wood-blocks and from movable type well over a hundred times before 1500. The small folio was part of a series which would train for 'Behaviour, gentle and devout', from manipulating a table knife to conducting a conversation, from the art of weeping and blowing your nose to the art of playing chess and dying.

[212] BALTRUSAITIS, Jurgis. *Le moyen âge fantastique. Antiquités et exotisme dans l'art gothique.* Paris, A. Colin, 1955.
[213] LUTHER, Martin. interpretation to Ps. 90 WA 40/III, 485 ff.

This was not a book of remote preparation for death through a virtuous life, nor a reminder to the reader of an inevitable steady decline of physical forces and the constant danger of death. It was a 'how to' book in the modern sense, a complete guide to the business of dying, a method to be learned while one was in good health and to be kept at one's fingertips for use in that inescapable hour. The book is not written for monks and ascetics but for 'carnall and secular' men for whom the ministrations of the clergy were not available. It served as a model for similar instructions, often written in a much less matter-of-fact spirit by people like Savonarola, Luther and Jeremy Taylor. Men felt responsible for the expression their face would show in death.[214]

As the decay of the body acquired a new finality, the first true portraits of Kings appear in European art, executed in order to render the individual atemporal personality of the deceased ruler present at his funeral. The humanists remembered their dead not as ghosts or souls, saints or symbols, but as continuing historical presences.[215]

In popular devotion a new kind of curiosity about the after-

[214] The response to 'natural' death was a profound transformation of behaviour at the hour of death. For contemporary literature see: O'CONNOR, Mary Catherine. *The art of dying well. The development of the Ars Moriendi.* New York, AMS Press, 1966. KLEIN, L. *Die Bereitung zum Sterben, Studien zu den evangelischen Sterbebüchern des 16. Jahrhunderts*, Diss. Göttingen, 1958. For customs see: BERGER, Placidus. *Religiöser Brauchtum im Umkreis der Sterbeliturgie in Deutschland*, in: Zeitschrift für Missionswissenschaft und Religionswissenschaft, V. 48, pp. 108–248. ARIES, Philippe. *La mort inversée. Le changement des attitudes devant la mort dans les sociétés occidentales*, in: Archives Européennes de Sociologie. Vol. VIII, No. 2, 1967, pp. 169–195, p. 175: '... L'homme du second moyen âge et de la Renaissance (par opposition a l'homme du premier moyen âge, de Roland, qui se survit chez les paysans de Tolstoï) tenait a participer à sa propre mort, parce qu'il voyait dans cette mort un moment exceptionnel où son individualité recevait sa forme definitive. Il n'était le maître de sa vie que dans la mesure où il était le maître de sa mort. Sa mort lui appartenait et à lui seul. Or, a partir du XVIIe siècle, il a cessé d'exercer seul sa souveraineté sur sa propre vie et, par conséquent, sur sa mort. Il l'a partagée avec sa famille. Auparavant sa famille était écartées des décisions graves qu'il devait prendre en vue de la mort, et qu'il prenait seul.' See also: BAMBECK, Manfred. *Tod und Unsterblichkeit. Studien zum Lebensgefühl der französischen Renaissance nach dem Werke Ronsarde.* (MS), 177, VI, Bl. Diss. Univ. Frankfurt am Main, 1954. REIFSCHNEIDER, Hildegard. *Die Vorstellung des Todes und des Jenseits in der geistlichen Literatur des XII Jh.* (MS)177, 76 Bl. Tübingen, Diss. 1948. KLASS, Eberhard. *Die Schilderung des Sterbens im mittelhochdeutschen Epos. Ein Beitrag zur mittelhochdeutschen Stilgeschichte.* Oderberg (Mark) 99 S. Diss. Univ. Greifswald, 1931.

[215] KUNSTLER, Gustav. *Das Bildnis Rudolf des Stifters, Herzogs von Österreich, und seine Funktion.* Excerpt from 'Mitteilungen der Österreichischen Galerie 1972' about the very first such portrait.

life developed. Fantastic horror stories about dead bodies and artistic representations of purgatory both multiplied.[216] The grotesque concern of the 17th century with ghosts and souls underscores the growing anxiety of a culture faced with the call of death rather than the judgement of God.[217] In many parts of the Christian world the dance of death became a standard decoration in the entrance of parish churches. The Spaniards brought the skeleton man to America, where he fused with the Aztec idol of death. Their Mestizo offspring,[218] on its rebound to Europe, influenced the face of death throughout the Hapsburg Empire from Holland to the Tyrol. After the Reformation European death became and remained macabre.

Simultaneously medical folk practices multiplied, all designed to help people to meet their death with dignity as individuals. New superstitious devices were developed so that one might recognize whether one's sickness required the acceptance of approaching death or some kind of treatment. If the flower thrown into the fountain of the sanctuary drowned, it was useless to spend money on remedies. People tried to be ready when death came, to have the steps well learnt for the last dance. Remedies against a painful agony multiplied, but most of them were still to be performed under the conscious direction of the dying who played a new role and played it consciously. Children could help a mother or father to die, but only if they did not hold them back by crying. A person was supposed to indicate when he wanted to be lowered from his bed onto the earth which would soon engulf him, and when the prayers were to start. But bystanders knew that they were to keep the doors open to make it easy for death to come, to avoid noise so as not to frighten death away, and finally to turn their eyes respectfully away from the dying man in

---

[216] VOVELLE, G. and M. *La mort et l'au-delà en Provence d'après les autels des âmes du purgatoire. XVe-XXe siècles*, in: Annals, Economies, Sociétés, Civilisations, 1969, pp. 1602–1634. PATCH, H. *The other world according to description in medieval literature.* Harvard 1950.

[217] For the 'judgement' in the history of religions see: SOURCES ORIENTALES. *Le jugement des morts.* Le Seuil, 1962. KRETZENBACHER, Leopold. *Die Seelenwaage. Zur religiösen Idee vom Jenseitsgericht auf der Schicksalwaage in Hochreligion*, Bildkunst und Volksglaube. 1958.

[218] FORSTER, Merlin H. editor. *La muerte en la poesía mexicana. Prólogo y selección de Merlin Forster.* Mexico, Editorial Diogenes, 1970. RODRIGUEZ MONEGAL, Emir. *Death as a key to Mexican reality in the works of Octavio Paz.* Yale Univ. mimeo.

order to leave him alone during this most personal event.[219]

Neither priest nor doctor were expected to assist the poor man in typical 15th- and 16th-century death. In principle, medical writers recognized two opposite services the physician could perform. He could either assist healing or help the coming of an easy and speedy death. It was his duty to recognize the 'facies Hippocratica',[220] the special traits which indicated that the patient was already in the grip of death. In healing, as in withdrawal, the doctor was anxious to work hand in glove with nature. The question as to whether medicine ever could 'prolong' life was heatedly disputed in the medical schools of Palermo, Fez, and even Paris. Many Arab and Jewish doctors denied this power outright, and declared such an attempt to interfere with the order of nature to be blasphemous.[221]

Vocational zeal tempered by philosophical resignation comes through clearly in the writings of Paracelsus.[222] 'Nature knows the boundaries of her course. According to her own appointed term, she confers upon each of her creatures its proper life span, so that its energies are consumed during the time that elapses between the moment of its birth and its predestined end . . . a man's death is nothing but the end of his daily work, an expiration of air, the consummation of his innate balsamic self-curing power, the extinction of the rational light of nature, and a great separation of the three: body, soul and spirit. Death is a return to the womb.' Without excluding transcendence, death has

---

[219] In rural areas these customs live on: VAN GENNEP, Arnold. *Manuel de folklore français contemporain*, first volume, I and II. *Du berceau à la tombe*. Paris, Picard, 1943/1946. KRISS-RETTENBECK, Lenz. *Tod und Heilserwartung*, in: Bilder und Zeichen religiösen Volksglaubens. München, Verlag Georg Callwey, 1963, pp. 49–56. See articles on Sterbegeläute, Sterben, Sterbender, Sterbekerze, Tod, Tod ansagen, Tote (der), Totenbahre, by GEIGER, Paulin: *Handwörterbuch des deutschen Aberglaubens*. Berlin 1936/1937, Vol. VIII. FREYBE, Albert. *Das alte deutsche Leichenmahl in seiner Art und Entartung*. 1909.

[220] SCHMID, Magnus. *Zum Phänomen der Leiblichkeit in der Antike dargstellt an der 'Facies Hippocratica'*, in: Sudhoff Arch., 1966, Beiheft 7, pp. 168–177. SUDHOFF, Karl. *Eine kleine deutsche Todesprognostik*, in: Arch. Gesch. Med. 1911, 5, p. 240. SUDHOFF, Karl. *Abermal eine deutsche Lebens- und Todesprognostik*, in: Arch. Gesch. Med. 1911, 6, p. 231.

[221] LEIBOWITZ, Joshua O. *A responsum of Maimonides concerning the termination of life*, in: Koroth. A quarterly Journal devoted to the History of Medicine and Science. Jerusalem, Vol. 5, 1–2, September, 1963.

[222] PARACELSUS. *Selected writings*. Transl. by Norbert Guterman. Princeton Univ. Press, Bollingen series XXVIII, 1969.

become a natural phenomenon, no longer requiring that blame be placed on some evil agent.

The new image of death helped to reduce the human body to an object. Up to this time, the corpse had been considered as something quite unlike other things: it was treated almost like a person. The law recognized its standing: the dead could sue and be sued by the living, and criminal proceedings against the dead were common. Pope Urban VIII, poisoned by his successor, was dug up, solemnly judged a simonist, had his right hand cut off, and was thrown into the Tiber. After being hanged as a thief, a man might still have his head cut off for being a traitor. The dead could also be called to witness. The widow could still repudiate her husband by putting the keys and his purse on his casket. Even today the executor acts in the name of the dead, and we still speak of the 'desecration' of a grave or the secularization of a public cemetery when it is turned into a park. The appearance of natural death was necessary for the corpse to be deprived of much of its legal standing.[223]

The arrival of natural death also prepared the way for new attitudes towards death and disease, which became common in the late 17th century. During the Middle Ages, the human body had been sacred; now the physician's scalpel had access to the corpse itself. Its dissection had been considered by the humanist Gerson to be 'a sacrilegious profanation, a useless cruelty exercised by the living against the dead'.[224] But at the same time that Everyman's Death began to emerge in person in the morality plays, the corpse first appears as a teaching object in the amphitheatre of the Renaissance university. When the first authorized public dissection took place in Montpellier in

[223] BRUNNER, Heinrich. *Deutsche Rechtsgeschichte*. Vol. I, Berlin, Von Duncker und Humbolt, 1961, esp. p. 254 ff. FISCHER, Paul. *Strafen und sichernde Massnahmen gegen Tote im germanischen und deutschen Recht*. Düsseldorf, 1936. FEHR, H. *Tod und Teufel im alten Recht*, in: Zeitschrift der Savigny Stiftung für Rechtsgeschichte, 67, Germ. Abt. 1950, pp. 50–75. GEIGER, Paul, *Leiche*, in: Handwörterbuch des deutschen Aberglaubens. Berlin, 1932/1933. Band V. KÖNIG, Karl. *Die Behandlung der Toten in Frankreich im späteren Mittelalter und zu Beginn der Neuzeit* (1350–1550). XVII, 94 S. (MS). Diss. Univ. Leipzig. 1921. HENTIG, Hans von. *Der nekrotrope Mensch: vom Totenglauben zur morbiden Totennähe*. Stuttgart, 1964. DOLL, Paul-J. *Les droits de la science après la mort*, in: Diogene, No. 75, July–September, 1971.

[224] BARIETY, Maurice, COURY, Charles. *La dissection*, in: Histoire de la médecine Paris, Fayard, 1963, pp. 409–411.

1375, this new learned activity was declared obscene, and the performance could not be repeated for several years. A generation later, permission was given for one corpse a year to be dissected within the borders of the German empire. At the University of Bologna, also, one body was dissected each year just before Christmas, and the ceremony was inaugurated by a procession, accompanied by exorcisms, and took three days. During the 15th century, the University of Lerida in Spain was entitled to the corpse of one criminal every three years, to be dissected in the presence of a notary assigned by the Inquisition. In England in 1540, the faculties of the universities were authorized to claim four corpses a year from the hangman. Attitudes changed so rapidly that by 1561 the Venetian Senate ordered the hangman to take instruction from Dr. Fallopius in order to provide him with corpses well suited for 'anatomizing'. Rembrandt painted 'Dr. Tulp's Lesson' in 1632. Public dissection became a favoured subject for paintings and, in the Netherlands, a common event at carnivals. The first step towards surgery on TV and in the movies had been taken. The physician had advanced his knowledge of anatomy and his power to exhibit his skill; but both were disproportionate to an advance in his ability to heal. Medical rituals helped to orient, repress or allay the fear and anguish generated by a death that had become macabre. The anatomy of Vesalius rivalled Holbein's *Danse Macabre* somewhat as scientific sex-guides now rival *Playboy* and *Penthouse* magazines.

Bourgeois Death

Baroque death counterpointed an aristocratically organized heaven.[225] The church vault might depict a last judgement with separate spaces reserved for savages, commoners and nobles, but the Dance of Death beneath depicted the mower, who used his scythe regardless of post or rank. Precisely because macabre equality belittled worldly privilege, it also made it more legiti-

[225] BAUER, Hermann. *Der Himmel im Rokoko: das Fresko im deutschen Kirchenraum im 18. Jahrhundert*, Pustet, 1965.

mate.[226] However, with the rise of the bourgeois family,[227] equality in death came to an end: those who could afford it began to pay to keep death away.

Francis Bacon was the first to speak about the prolongation of life as a new task for physicians. He divided medicine into three offices: 'First, the preservation of health, second, the cure of disease, and third, the prolongation of life,' and extolled the 'third part of medicine, regarding the prolongation of life: this is a new part, and deficient, although the most noble of all'. The medical profession did not even consider facing this task, until, some one hundred and fifty years later, there appeared a host of clients who were anxious to pay them to try. This was a new type of rich man who refused to die in retirement and insisted on being carried away by death from natural exhaustion while still on the job. He refused to accept death unless he was in good health in an active old age. Montaigne had already ridiculed such people as exceptionally conceited: ' 'Tis the last and extreme form of dying . . . what an idle conceit is it to expect to die of a decay of strength which is the effect of the extremest age, and to propose to ourselves no shorter lease on life . . . as if it were contrary to nature to see a man break his neck with a fall, be drowned by shipwreck, be snatched away with pleurisy or the plague . . . we

[226] Reflection of death in 17th and 18th century literature: SEXAU, Richard, Der Tod in deutschen Drama des 17. und 18. Jahrhunderts (von Griphius bis. zum Sturm and Drang.) Berlin, 1906. Volkständige Dissertation, No. 9 von 'Untersuchungen zur neueren Sprach- und Literatur Geschichte'. Bern. 1907. WENTZLAFF-EGGEBERT, Friedrich-Wilhelm. Das Problem des Todes in der deutschen Lyrik des 17. Jahrhunderts. Erster Hauptteil und Schluss Palaestra 171. Untersuchungen und Texte aus der deutschen und englischen Philologie. Leipzig, 1931. THOMPSON, W. M. Der Tod in der englische Lyrik des 17. Jahrhunderts. Breslau, 1935.

[227] ARIES, Philippe. La mort inversée. Le changement des attitudes devant la mort dans les sociétés occidentales, in: Archives Européennes de Sociologie. Vol. VIII, No. 2, 1967. pp. 169-195. This article was recently translated into English by Bernard Murchland in Hastings Center Studies, May 1974, Vol. 2, No. 2, as Death inside out.: '. . . in the late Middle Ages (in opposition to the first Middle Ages, the age of Roland, which lives on in the peasants of Tolstoï) and the Renaissance, a man insisted upon participating in his own death because he saw in it an exceptional moment—a moment which gave his individuality its definitive form. He was only the master of his life to the extent that he was the master of his death. His death belonged to him, and to him alone. From the 17th century onward, one began to abdicate sole sovereignty over life, as well as over death. These matters came to be shared with the family which had previously been excluded from the serious decisions; all decisions had been made by the dying person, alone and with full knowledge of his impending death.' (Quoted in French, footnote 214.)

ought to call natural death that which is general, common and universal.'[228] Such people were few in his time; by 1830 their numbers had increased. The preacher expecting to go to heaven, the philosopher denying the existence of the soul, and the merchant wanting to see his capital double once more, were all in agreement that the only death that accorded with nature was one which would overtake them at their desks.[229]

There was no evidence to show that the age-specific life expectancy of most people in their sixties had increased by the middle of the 18th century, but there is no doubt that new technology had made it possible for the old and rich to hang on while doing what they had done in middle age. The pampered could stay on the job because their living and working conditions had eased. The Industrial Revolution had begun to create employment opportunities for the weak, sickly and old. Sedentary work, hitherto rare, had come into its own.[230] Rising entrepreneurship and capitalism favoured the boss who had had the time to accumulate capital and experience. Roads had improved: a general affected by gout could now command a battle from his wagon, and decrepit diplomats could travel from London to Vienna or Moscow. Centralized nation states increased the need for scribes and an enlarged bourgeoisie. The new and small class of old men had a greater chance of survival because their lives at home, on the street, and at work had become physically less demanding. Aging had become a way of capitalizing life. Years at the desk, either at the counter or the school bench, began to bear interest on the market. The young of the middle class, whether gifted or not, were now for the first time sent to school thus allowing the old to stay on the job. The bourgeoisie who

[228] *Essays*, Book I, Chapter 57.

[228] PEIGNOT, G. *Choix de testaments anciens et modernes, remarquables par leur importance, leur singularité ou leur bizarrerie.* 2 vols., Paris, Renouard, 1929. VOVELLE, Michel. *Mourir autrefois. Attitudes collectives devant la mort aux XVIIe et XVIIIe siècles.* Paris, Archives Gallimard-Julliard, 1974. VOVELLE, Michel. *Piété baroque et déchristianisation en Provence au XVIIIe siècle: les attitudes devant la mort d'après les clauses des testaments.* Paris, Plon, 1974. POLLOCK and MAITLAND. *The last will,* in: The history of English law. Cambridge Univ. Press, 1968. Vol. 2, Chap. VI, pp. 314–356.

[230] ARIES, Philippe. *Les techniques de la mort,* in: Histoire des populations françaises et de leurs attitudes devant la vie depuis le XVIIIe siècle. Paris, Seuil, 1971, p. 373. (first edition 1948).

could afford to eliminate 'social death' by avoiding retirement, created 'childhood' to keep their young under control.[231]

Along with the economic status of the old, the value of their bodily functions increased. In the 16th century a 'young wife is death to an old man', and in the 17th 'old men who play with young maids dance with death'. At the court of Louis XIV the old lecher was a laughing stock; by the time of the Congress of Vienna he had turned into an object of envy. To die while courting one's grandson's mistress became wishful thinking.

A new myth about the social value of the old was developed. Primitive hunters, gatherers and nomads had usually killed them, and peasants had put them into the back room,[232] but now the patriarch appeared as a literary ideal. Wisdom was attributed to him just because of his age. It first became tolerable and then appropriate that the elderly should attend with solicitude to the rituals deemed necessary to keep up their tottering bodies. No physician was yet in attendance to take on this task, which lay beyond the competence claimed by apothecary or herbalist, barber or surgeon, university-trained doctor or travelling quack. But it was this peculiar demand that helped to create a new kind of self-styled healer.[233]

[231] ARIES, Philippe. *L'enfant et la vie familiale sous l'ancien régime*. Paris, Plon, 1960, chap. II, p. 23 ff. Engl. title: *Centuries of childhood*, Cape.

[232] Killing the aged was a widespread custom until recent times. KOTY, John. *Die Behandlung der Alten und Kranken bei den Naturvölkern*, 1934. (Forschgn. z. Völkerpsychologie und Soziologie, Hrag. v. Thurnwald 13.) PEUCKERT, Will-Eich. Ed. *Altentötung*, in: Handwörterbuch der Sage. Namens des Verbandes der Vereine für Volkskunde. Göttingen, Vandenhoeck and Ruprecht, 1961. WISSE, J. *Selbstmord und Todesfurcht bei den Naturvölkern*. Zutphen, 1933. Infanticide remained important enough to influence population trends until the 9th century. COLEMAN, Emily R. *L'infanticide dans le haut moyen age*. Translated from the English by A. Chamoux, in: Annales. Economies, Sociétés, Civilisations. Paris, Armand Colin, No. 2, March-April 1974. pp. 315–335.

[233] ACKERKNECHT, Erwin H. *Death in the history of medicine*, in: Bulletin of the History of Medicine. Vol. 42, 1968. Death remained a marginal problem in medical literature from the old Greeks until Giovanni Maria Lancisi (1654–1720) during the first decade of the eighteenth century. Then quite suddenly the 'signs of death' acquired extraordinary importance. Apparent death became a major evil feared by the Enlightenment. AUGENER, Margot. *Scheintod als medizinisches Problem im 18. Jahrhundert*, in: Mitteilungen zur Geschichte der Medizin. Kiel, Nos 6 and 7, 1967. The same philosophers who were the minority which positively denied the survival of a soul, also developed a secularized fear of hell which might threaten them if they were buried while only apparently dead. Philanthropists fighting for those in danger of apparent death founded societies dedicated to the succour of the drowning or burning, and tests were developed for making sure that they had died. THOMSON,

Formerly, only King and Pope had been under an obligation to remain in command until the day of his death. They alone consulted the faculties: the Arabs from Salerno in the Middle Ages, or the Renaissance men from Padua or Montpellier. Kings kept court physicians to do what barbers did for the commoner: bleed them and purge them, and in addition, protect them from poisons. Kings neither set out to live longer than others, nor expected their personal physicians to give special dignity to their declining years. In contrast, the new class of old men saw in death the absolute price for absolute economic value.[234] The aging accountant wanted a doctor who would drive away death; when the end approached, he wanted to be formally 'given up' by his doctor and be served his last repast with the special bottle reserved for the occasion. The role of the valetudinarian was thereby created and, with it, the economic power of the contemporary physician.

The ability to survive longer, the refusal to retire before death, and the demand for medical assistance in an incurable condition had joined forces to give rise to a new concept of sickness: the type of health to which old age could aspire. In the years just before the French Revolution this had become the health of the rich and the powerful; within a generation chronic disease became fashionable for the young and pretentious, consumptive features[235] the sign of premature wisdom, and the need for travel into warm climates a claim to genius. Medical care for protracted ailments, even though they might lead to untimely death, had become a mark of distinction.

Elisabeth. *The role of the physician in human societies of the 18th century*, in: Bull. Hist. Medicine, 37, 1963, pp. 43–51. One of these tests consisted of blowing with a trumpet into the dead man's ear. The hysteria about apparent death disappeared with the French Revolution as suddenly as it had appeared at the dawn of the century. Doctors began to be concerned with reanimation a century before they were employed in the hope of prolonging the life of the old. See also: STEINGIESSER, Hildegard. *Was die Ärzte aller Zeiten vom Sterben wussten*. Arbeiten der deutsch-nordischen Gesellschaft für Geschichte der Medizin, der Zahnheilkunde und der Naturwissenschaften. Univ. Verlag Ratsbuchhandlung L. Bamberg, Greifswald, 1936.
[234] ADORNO, Theodor W. *Minima Moralia. Reflexionen aus dem beschädigten Leben*. Suhrkamp, 1970.
[235] EBSTEIN, E. *Die Lungenschwindsucht in der Weltliteratur*. Zs. f. Bücherfreunde, 5, 1913. WEISFERT, J. N. *Das Problem des Schwindsuchtskranken in Drama und Roman*, in: Deutscher Journalistenspiegel, 3, 1927.

By contrast, a reverse judgement now could be made on the ailments of the poor, and the ills from which they had always died could be defined as untreated sickness. It did not matter at all if the treatment doctors could provide for these ills had any effect on the progress of the sickness; the lack of such treatment began to mean that they were condemned to die an unnatural death, an idea that fitted the bourgeois' image of the poor as un-educated and unproductive. From now on the ability to die a 'natural' death was reserved to one social class: those who could afford to die as patients.

Health became the privilege of waiting for timely death, no matter what medical service was needed for this purpose. In an earlier epoch, death had carried the hour glass. In woodcuts, both skeleton and onlooker grin when the victim refuses death. Now the middle class seized the clock and employed doctors to tell death when to strike. The Enlightenment attributed a new power to the doctor, without being able to verify whether or not he had acquired any new influence over the outcome of dangerous sickness.

Clinical Death

The French Revolution marked a short interruption in the medicalization of death. Its ideologues believed that untimely death would not strike in a society built on its triple ideal. But the opening of the doctor's clinical eye caused him to look at death in a new perspective. Whereas the merchants of the 18th century had determined the outlook on death with the help of the charlatans they employed and paid, now the clinicians began to shape the public's vision. We have seen death turn from God's call into a 'natural' event and later into a 'force of nature'; in a further mutation it is now turned into an 'untimely' event unless coming to those who were both healthy and old. Now it had become the outcome of specific diseases certified by the doctor.

Death has paled into a metaphorical figure, and killer diseases have taken his place. The general force of nature that had been celebrated as 'death' turned into a host of specific causations of clinical demise. Many 'deaths' now roam the world. A number of book plates from private libraries of late 19th-century physicians show the doctor battling with personified diseases at the bedside of his patient. The hope of doctors to control the outcome of specific diseases gave rise to the myth that they had power over death. The new powers attributed to the profession gave rise to the new status of the clinician.

While the city physician became a clinician, the country physician became first sedentary and then a member of the local élite. At the time of the French Revolution he had still belonged to the travelling folk. The surplus of army surgeons from the Napoleonic wars came home with a vast experience and looked for a living. Military men trained on the battlefield, they soon became the first resident healers in France, Italy and Germany. The simple people did not quite trust their techniques and staid burghers were shocked by their rough ways, but still they found clients because of their competence as medics. They sent their sons to the new medical schools springing up in the cities, and these upon their return created the role of the country doctor which remained unchanged up to the time of World War II. They derived a steady income from playing the family doctor to the middle class who could well afford them. A few of the city or town rich acquired prestige by living as patients of famous clinicians, but in the early 19th century a much more serious competition for the town doctor still came from the medical technicians of old—the midwife, the tooth-puller, the veterinarian, the barber and sometimes the public nurse. Notwithstanding the newness of his role and resistance to it from above and below, the European country doctor, by mid-century, had become a member of the middle class. He earned enough from playing lackey to a squire, was family friend to other notables, paid occasional visits to the lowly sick and sent his complicated cases to his clinical colleague in town. While 'timely' death had originated in the emerging class consciousness of the bourgeois, 'clinical' death originated in the emerging professional consciousness of the new, scientifically-trained doctor. Henceforth, a timely death with clinical symptoms became the ideal of middle-class doctors, and it was soon to become incorporated into the social goal of trade unions.

Trade Union Claims to a Natural Death

In our century, a valetudinarian's death while undergoing treatment by clinically trained doctors came to be perceived, for the first time, as a civil right. Old age medical care was written into union contracts. The capitalist privilege of natural extinction from exhaustion in a director's chair gave way to the proletarian demand for health services during retirement. The bourgeois hope of continuing as a dirty old man in the office was ousted by the dream of an active sex life on social security in a retirement village. Lifelong care for every clinical condition soon became a peremptory demand for access to a natural death. Lifelong institutional medical care had become a service that society owed all its members.

'Natural death' now appeared in dictionaries. One major German encyclopedia published in 1909 defines it by means of contrast: 'abnormal death is opposed to natural death because it results from sickness, violence, or mechanical and chronic disturbances'. A reputable dictionary of philosophical concepts states that 'natural death comes without previous sickness, without definable specific cause'. It was this macabre yet hallucinating death-concept that became intertwined with the concept of social progress. Legally valid claims to equality in clinical death disseminated the contradictions of bourgeois individualism among the working class. The right to a natural death was formulated as a claim to equal consumption of medical services, rather than as a freedom from the evils of industrial work or as new liberties and powers for self-care. This unionized concept of an 'equal clinical death' is thus the inverse of the ideal proposed in the National Assembly of Paris in 1792: it is a deeply medicalized ideal.

First of all, this new image of death endorses new levels of social control. Society has become responsible for preventing each man's death: treatment, effective or not, can be made into a duty. Any fatality occurring without medical treatment is liable to become a coroner's case. The encounter with a doctor becomes almost as inexorable as the encounter with death. I know of a woman who tried, unsuccessfully, to kill herself. She was brought to the hospital in a coma, with two bullets lodged in her spine.

Using heroic measures the surgeon kept her alive and considers her case a double success: she lives, and she is totally paralysed so that he no longer has to worry about her ever attempting suicide again.

Our new image of death also befits the industrial ethos. The good death has irrevocably become that of the standard consumer of medical care. Just as at the turn of the century all men were defined as pupils, born into original stupidity and standing in need of eight years of schooling before they could enter productive life, today they are stamped from birth as patients who need all kinds of treatment if they want to lead life the right way. Just as compulsory educational consumption came to be used as a device to discriminate at work, so medical consumption became a device to alleviate unhealthy work, dirty cities, and nerve-racking transportation.[236] What need is there to worry about a less murderous environment when doctors are industrially equipped to act as life savers!

Finally, 'death under compulsory care' encourages the re-emergence of the most primitive delusions about the causes of death. As we have seen, primitive people do not die of their own death, they do not carry finitude in their bones, and they are still close to the subjective immortality of the beast. Among them, death always requires a supernatural explanation, somebody to blame: the curse of an enemy, the spell of a magician, the breaking of the yarn in the hands of the Parsee, or God dispatching his angel of death. In the dance with his mirror image, European death emerged as an event independent of another's will, an inexorable force of nature that all had to face on their own. The imminence of death was an exquisite and constant reminder of the fragility and tenderness of life. During the late Middle Ages, the discovery of 'natural' death became one of the mainsprings of European lyric and drama. But the same imminence of death, once perceived as an extrinsic threat coming from nature, became a major challenge for the emerging engineer. If the civil engineer had learned to manage earth, and the pedagogue-become-educator to manage knowledge, why should the

[236] GIEDION, Siegfried. *Mechanization takes command: a contribution to anonymous history.* New York, Norton, 1969. 743 p. On mechanization and death see pp. 209–240.

biologist–physician not manage death? When the doctor contrived to step between humanity and death, the latter lost the immediacy and intimacy he had gained four hundred years earlier.

The change in the doctor–death relationship can be well illustrated by following the iconographic treatment of this theme.[237] In the age of the Dance of Death, the physician is rare; in the only picture I have located in which death treats the doctor as a colleague, he has taken an old man by one hand, while in the other he carries a glass of urine, and seems to be asking the physician to confirm his diagnosis. In the age of the Dance of Death, the skeleton man makes the doctor the main butt of his jokes. In the earlier period, while death still wore some flesh, he asks the doctor to confirm in the latter's own mirror image what he thought he knew about man's innards. Later, as a fleshless skeleton, he teases the doctor about his impotence, jokes about or rejects his honoraria, offers medicine as pernicious as that which the physician dispensed, and treats the doctor as just one more common mortal by snatching him into the dance. Baroque death seems to intrude constantly into the doctor's activities, making fun of him while he sells his wares at a fair, interrupting his consultations, transforming his medicine bottles into hour glasses, or taking the doctor's place on a visit to the pesthouse. In the 18th century a new motif appears: teasing the physician because of his pessimistic diagnosis and death seems to enjoy abandoning those sick persons whom the doctor has condemned. Until the 19th century, death deals always with the doctor or with the sick, usually taking the initiative in the action. The contestants are at opposite ends of the sick bed. Only after clinical sickness and clinical death had developed considerably do we find the first pictures in which the doctor assumes the initiative and interposes himself between his patient and death. We have to wait until after World War I before we see physicians wrangling with the skeleton, tearing a young woman from its embrace, and wresting the scythe from death's hand. By 1930 a smiling white-coated man is rushing against a whimpering skeleton and crushing it like a fly with two volumes of Marle's *Lexicon of Therapy*. In other pictures, the doctor raises one hand and bans

[237] especially BLOCK, Werner; WARTHIN, Alfred Scott and BRIESENMEISTER, Dietrich. See footnote 210.

death while holding up the arms of a young woman whom death grips by the feet. Max Klinger represents the physician clipping the feathers of a winged giant. Others show the physician locking the skeleton into prison or even kicking its bony bottom. Now the doctor rather than the patient struggles with death. As in primitive cultures, somebody can again be blamed when death triumphs; again, this somebody has no face, but he does hold a charter: the person is not a person but a class.

Today, when defence against death is included in social security, the culprit lurks within society. The culprit might be the class enemy who deprives the worker of sufficient medical care, the doctor who refuses to make a night visit, the multinational concern that raises the price of medicine, the capitalist or revisionist government that has lost control over its medicine men, or the administrator who partly trains physicians at the University of Delhi and then drains them off to London. The witchhunt traditional at the death of a tribal chief is being modernized. For every premature or clinically unnecessary death, somebody or some body can be found who irresponsibly delayed or prevented a medical intervention.

Much of the progress of social legislation during the first half of the 20th century would have been impossible without the revolutionary use of such an industrially graven death image. Neither the support necessary to agitate for such legislation, nor guilt feelings strong enough to enforce its enactment could have been aroused. But the claim to equal medical nurturing towards an equal kind of death has also served to consolidate the dependence of our contemporaries on a limitlessly expanding industrial system.

Death under Intensive Care

We cannot fully understand the deeply rooted structure of our social organization unless we see in it a multi-faceted exorcism of all forms of evil death. Our major institutions constitute a gigantic defence programme waging war on behalf of 'humanity' against death-dealing agencies and classes.[238] This is a total war. Not only

[238] KALISH, Richard A. *Death and dying. A briefly annotated bibliography*, in: BRIM, Orville. et al., editors. *The dying patient*. New York, Russel Sage Foundation,

medicine but also welfare, international relief, and development programmes are enlisted in this struggle. Ideological bureaucracies of all colours join the crusade. Revolution, repression, and even civil and international wars are justified in order to defeat the dictators or capitalists who can be blamed for the wanton creation and tolerance of sickness and death.[239]

Curiously, death became the enemy to be defeated at precisely the moment in which mega-death comes upon the scene. Not only the image of 'unnecessary' death is new, but also our image of the end of the world.[240] Death, the end of *my* world, and apocalypse, the end of *the* world, are intimately related; our attitude towards both has clearly been deeply affected by the atomic situation. The apocalypse has ceased to be just a mythological conjecture and has become a real contingency. Instead of being due to the will of God, or man's guilt, or the laws of nature, Armageddon has become a possible consequence of man's direct

---

1970, pp. 327–380, a bibliographic survey on English language literature on dying, limited mainly to items which deal with contemporary professional activity and, technology. SOLLITO, Sharmon, VEATCH, Robert. *Bibliography of society, ethics and the life sciences*. The Hastings Center, 1973, evaluates such activities from an ethical point of view. MCKNIGHT. A bibliography of 225 items of suggested readings for a course on death in modern society in a theological perspective. 10 pages, mineo lists contemporary Christian writings on death in an industrial society. KUTSCHER, Austin H. Jr. and KUTSCHER, Austin H. *A bibliography of books on death, bereavement, loss and grief*: 1935–1968. New York, Health Sciences Publishing Corp. 1969. EUTHANASIA EDUCATIONAL FUND. *Euthanasia: an annotated bibliography*. New York, 250 West 57th street, NY 10019. RILEY, John Jr. and HABENSTEIN, Robert W. *Death. 1. Death and bereavement. 2. the social organization of death*, in: International Encyclopedia of the Social Sciences. Macmillan, Vol. 4, 1968.

[239] FUCHS, Werner, footnote 200 denies that death is repressed in modern society. GORER, Geoffrey. *Death, grief and mourning*. New York, Doubleday, 1965. Gorer's thesis that death has taken the place of sex as the principal taboo seems to Fuchs unfounded and misleading. The thesis of death-repression is usually promoted by people of profoundly anti-industrial persuasions for the purpose of demonstrating the ultimate powerlessness of the industrial enterprise in the face of death. Talk about death-repression is used with insistence to construct apologies in favour of God and the afterlife. The fact that people have to die is taken as proof that they will never autonomously control reality. Fuchs interprets all theories which deny the quality of death as relics of a primitive past. He considers as scientific only those corresponding to his idea of a modern social structure. His image of contemporary death is a result of his study of the language used in German obituaries. He believes that what is called the 'repression' of death is due to a lack of effective acceptance of the increasingly more general belief in death as an unquestionable and final end.

[240] The irrational approach of a society dealing with death is reflected in the society's inability to deal with apocalypse. KOCH, Klaus. *Ratlos vor der Apokalyptik*. Gütersloh, Gütersloher Verlaghaus Gerd Mohn, 1970.

decision. An uncanny analogy exists between atomic and cobalt bombs: both are deemed necessary for the good of mankind, both are effective in providing man with power over the end. Medicalized social rituals represent one aspect of social control by means of the self-frustrating war against death.

Malinowski[241] has argued that death among primitive people threatens the cohesion and therefore the survival of the whole group. It triggers an explosion of fear and irrational expressions of defence. Group solidarity is saved by making out of the natural event a social ritual. The death of a member thereby becomes an occasion for an exceptional celebration.

The dominance of industry has disrupted and often dissolved most traditional bonds of solidarity. The impersonal rituals of Industrialized Medicine create an ersatz unity of mankind. They relate all its members to an identical pattern of 'desirable' death by proposing hospital death as the goal of economic development. The myth of progress of all people towards the same kind of death diminishes the feeling of guilt on the part of the 'haves' by transforming the ugly deaths of which 'have nots' die into the result of present underdevelopment, which ought to be remedied by further expansion of medical institutions.

Of course, medicalized[242] death has a different function in highly industrialized societies than it has in mainly rural nations. Within an industrial society, medical intervention in everyday life does not change the prevailing image of health and death, but rather caters to it. It diffuses the death image of the medicalized élite to the masses and reproduces it for future generations. But when 'death prevention' is applied outside of a cultural context in which consumers religiously prepare themselves for hospital deaths, the growth of hospital-based medicine inevitably constitutes a form of imperialist intervention. A socio-political image of death is imposed; people are deprived of their traditional vision of what constitutes health and death. The self-image that gives cohesion to their culture is dissolved, and

[241] MALINOWSKI, Bronislav. *Death and the reintegration of the group*, in: Magic, science and religion. New York, Doubleday, 1949, pp. 47–53.

[242] CASSEL, Eric J. *Dying in a technical society*, in: Hastings Center Studies,Vol. 2, No. 2, May 1974, pp. 31–36. 'There has been a shift of death from within the moral order to the technical order . . . I do not believe that men were inherently more moral in the past when the moral order predominated over the technical.'

atomized individuals can be incorporated into an international mass of highly 'socialized' health consumers. The expectation of medicalized death hooks the rich on unlimited insurance payments and lures the poor into a gilded deathtrap. The contradictions of bourgeois individualism are corroborated by the inability of people to die with any possibility of a realistic attitude towards death.[243] The Customs man guarding the frontier of Upper Volta with Mali explained to me this importance of death in relation to health. I wanted to know from him how people along the Niger could understand each other, though almost each village spoke a different tongue. For him this had nothing to do with language: 'As long as people cut the prepuce of their boys the way we do, and die our death, we can understand them well.'

In many a village in Mexico I have seen what happens when social security arrives. For a generation people continue in their traditional beliefs; they know how to deal with death, dying and grief. The new nurse and the doctor, thinking they know better, teach them about a Pantheon of evil clinical deaths, each one of which can be banned, at a price. Instead of modernizing people's skills for self-care, they preach the ideal of hospital death. By their ministration they urge the peasants to an unending search for the good death of international description, a search which will keep them consumers for ever.

Like all other major rituals of industrial society, medicine in practice takes the form of a game. The chief function of the physician becomes that of an umpire. He is the agent or representative of the social body, with the duty to make sure that everyone plays the game according to the rules.[244] The rules,

[243] MORIN, Edgar. *L'homme et la mort*. Paris, Seuil, 1970, who develops the argument.

[244] Industrialized humanity needs therapy from crib to terminal ward. A new kind of terminal therapist is suggested by KUBLER-ROSS, Elisabeth. *On death and dying* New York, Macmillan, 1969. The author suggests that the dying pass through several typical stages, and that appropriate treatment can ease this process for well-managed 'morituri'. RAMSEY, Paul. *The indignity of 'death with dignity'*, in: Hastings Center Studies, Vol. 2, No. 2, May 1974, pp. 47–62. There is a growing agreement among moralists in the early seventies that death has again to be accepted and all that can be done for the dying is to keep company with them in their final passage. But beneath this accord there is an increasing mundane, naturalistic and anti-humanistic interpretation of human life. MORISON, Robert S. *The last poem: the dignity of the inevitable and necessary. Commentary on Paul Ramsey*, in: Hastings

of course, forbid leaving the game and dying in any fashion which has not been specified by the umpire. Death no longer occurs except as the self-fulfilling prophecy of the medicine man.[245]

Through the medicalization of death, health care has become a monolithic world religion[246] whose tenets are taught in compulsory schools and whose ethical rules are applied to a bureaucratic restructuring of the environment: sex became a subject in the syllabus and sharing one's spoon is discouraged for the sake of hygiene. The struggle against death, which dominates the lifestyle of the rich, is translated by development agencies into a set of rules by which the poor of the earth shall be forced to conduct themselves.

Only a culture that evolved in highly industrialized societies could possibly have called forth the commercialization of the death image that I have just described. In its extreme form, 'natural death' is now that point at which the human organism

Center Studies, Vol. 2, No. 2, May 1974, pp. 62–66. Morison criticizes Ramsey who suggests that anyone unable to speak as a Christian ethicist must do so as some 'hypothetical common denominator'.

[245] LESTER, David. *Voodoo death: some new thoughts on an old phenomenon*, in: American Anthropologist, 74, 1972, pp. 386–390.

[246] DELOOZ, Pierre. *Who believes in the hereafter*, in: Godin, André, editor. Death and presence. Brussels, Lumen Vitae Press, 1972, pp. 17–38, shows that contemporary French public speakers have effectively separated belief in God from belief in the hereafter. DANBLON, Paul, GODIN, André. *How do people speak of death?*, in: Godin, André, editor, ibid, pp. 39–62. Danblon studied interviews with 60 French-speaking public figures. The cross-denominational analogies in their expressions, feelings and attitudes towards death are much stronger than their differences due to varying religious beliefs or practices. FLETCHER, Joseph F. *Antidysthanasia: the problem of prolonging death*, in: The Journal of Pastoral Care, Vol. XVIII, 1964, pp. 77–84, argues against the irresponsible prolongation of life, written from the point of view of a hospital chaplain, 'I would myself agree with Pius XII and with at least two Archbishops of Canterbury, Lang and Fisher, who have addressed themselves to this question, that the doctor's technical knowledge and his "educated guesses" and experience should be the basis for deciding the question as to whether there is any "reasonable hope". That determination is outside a layman's competence . . . But having determined that the condition is hopeless, I cannot agree that it is either prudent or fair to physicians as a fraternity to saddle them with the onus of alone deciding whether to let the patient go.' The thesis is common. It shows how even churches support professional judgement. This practical convergence of Christian and medical practice is in stark opposition to the attitude towards death in Christian theology. BOROS, Ladislaus. *Mysterium mortis. Der Mensch in der letzten Entscheidung*. Freiburg/Br., Walter Verlag, 1962. RAHNER, Karl. *Zur Theologie des Todes*. Herder, Freiburg, 1963.

refuses any further input of treatment. People[247] die when the electroencephalogram indicates that their brainwaves have flattened out: they do not take a last breath, or die because their heart stops. Socially approved death happens when man has become useless not only as a producer but also as a consumer. It is the point at which a consumer, trained at great expense, must finally be written off as a total loss. Death has become the ultimate form of consumer resistance.[248]

Traditionally the person best protected from death was the one whom society had condemned to die. Society felt threatened that the man on Death Row might use his tie to hang himself. Authority might be challenged if he took his life before the appointed hour. Today, the man best protected against setting the stage for his own dying is the sick person in critical condition. Society, acting through the medical system, decides when and after what indignities and mutilations he shall die.[249] The medicalization of society has brought the epoch of natural death to an end. Western man has lost the right to preside at his act of

[247] MAGUIRE, Daniel. *The freedom to die.* By working creatively, and in ways as yet unthought of, the lobby of the dying and the gravely ill could become a healing force in society, in: Commonweal, 11 August, 1972, pp. 423–428. ROBITSCHER, Jonas B. *The right to die. Do we have a right not to be treated?*, in: The Hastings Center Report, Vol. 2, No. 4, September, 1972, pp. 11–44.

[248] BRIM, Orville, FREEMAN, Howard, LEVINE, Sol, SCOTCH, Norman, editors *The dying patient.* New York, Russel Sage Foundation, 1960. They first deal with the spectrum of technical analysis and decision-making in which health professionals engage when they are faced with the task of determining the circumstances under which an individual's death should occur. They provide a series of recommendations about what might be done to make this engineered process 'somewhat less graceless and less distasteful for the patient, his family and most of all, the attending personnel'. In this anthology the macabre turns into a new kind of professionally conducted obscenity. See also: SUDNOW, David. *Dying in a public hospital*, in: BRIM, Orville et al., ibid, pp. 191–208.

[249] SUDNOW, David, ibid, in his study of the social organization reports: '. . . a nurse was observed spending two or three minutes trying to close the eyelids of a woman patient. The nurse explained that the woman was dying. She was trying to get the lids to remain in a closed position. After several unsuccessful attempts, the nurse got them shut and said, with a sigh of accomplishment, "Now they're right." When questioned about what she was doing, she said that a patient's eyes must be closed after death, so that the body will resemble a sleeping person. It was more difficult to accomplish this, she explained, after the muscles and skin had begun to stiffen. She always tried, she said, to close them *before* death. This made for greater efficiency when it came time for ward personnel to wrap the body. It was a matter of consideration towards those workers who preferred to handle dead bodies as little as possible.' pp. 192–193.

dying. Health, or the autonomous power to cope, has been expropriated down to the last breath. Technical death has won its victory over dying.[250] Mechanical death has conquered and destroyed all other deaths.

[250] BRILLAT-SAVARIN. *Méditation XXVI, de la mort*, in: Physiologie du gout. Brillat-Savarin attended his 93-year-old great-aunt when she was dying. 'She had kept all her faculties and one would not have noticed her state but for her smaller appetite and her feeble voice. "Are you there, nephew?" "Yes aunt, I am at your service and I think it would be a good idea if you had some of this lovely old wine." "Give it to me, my friend, liquids always go down." I made her swallow half a glass of my best wine. She perked up immediately and turning her once beautiful eyes towards me. She said: "Thank you for this last favour. If you ever get to my age you will see that death becomes as necessary as sleep." These were her last words and half an hour later she was asleep for ever.'

PART 4
THE POLITICS OF HEALTH

9 THE RECOVERY OF HEALTH

MUCH suffering has always been man-made. Records of this intentional harassment of man by man have been kept. History is one long catalogue of enslavement and exploitation, usually told in the epics of conquerors or sung in the elegies of the victims. War was at the heart of this tale, with the pillage, the famine and the pestilence that came in its wake. War between commonwealths and classes has been until recently the main agency of man-made misery. Now the unwanted physical, social and psychological side-effects of so-called peaceful enterprises compete in destructive power with those of war, and statistics are faithfully kept.

Man is the only animal whose evolution has been conditioned by adaptation on more than one front. If he did not succumb to predators and forces of nature he had to cope with use and abuse by others of his own kind. In this struggle with the elements and with his neighbour, his character and culture were formed, and his instincts withered.

Animals adapt through evolution in response to changes in their natural environment. Only in man can challenge become conscious and his response to difficult persons and threatening situations take the form of rational action and of conscious habit. Man can plan his relations to nature and neighbour, and he can survive even when his enterprise has partly failed. He is the animal who can patiently endure trials and learn by understanding them. He is the sole being who can and must resign himself to limits when he becomes aware of them. A conscious response to painful sensations, to impairment and to eventual death is part of man's coping ability. The capacity for revolt and perseverance, for patience and resignation, are integral parts of human health.

But nature and neighbour are only two of the three frontiers at which man must cope. A third front on which doom can threaten has always been recognized. Man must survive his dream which myth has both shaped and controlled. Society must cope with the irrational desires of its members. To date, myth has fulfilled the function of assuring the common man that he is safe on this third frontier if his action is kept within bounds. Disaster only threatens those few who try to outwit the gods. The common man perishes from infirmity or from violence. Only the rebel against the human condition falls prey to Nemesis, the envy of the gods.

Industrialized Nemesis

Prometheus was hero, not Everyman. Driven by radical greed (pleonexia), he trespassed the measures of man (aitia and mesotes) and in unbounded presumption (hubris) stole fire from heaven. He thus inevitably brought Nemesis on himself. He was put into irons and welded to a Caucasian rock. A vulture preyed all day at his innards, and heartlessly healing gods kept him alive by regrafting his liver each night. Nemesis inflicted on him a kind of pain meant for demi-gods, not for men. His hopeless and unending suffering turned the hero into an immortal reminder of inescapable cosmic retaliation.

The social nature of Nemesis has now changed. With the industrialization of desire and the engineering of ritual responses hubris has spread. Unbounded material progress has become Everyman's goal. Industrial hubris has destroyed the mythical framework of limits to irrational fantasies. Engineering has materialized the myth, has made technical answers to mad dreams seem rational, and has turned the pursuit of destructive values into a conspiracy between purveyor and client. Nemesis for the masses is now the inescapable backlash of industrial progress. It is the material monster born from the over-reaching industrial dream. It has spread as far and as wide as universal schooling, mass transportation, industrial wage-labour and the medicalization of health. The winged goddess of nature's self-defence now comes to us through the networks of TV, highways, supermarkets and clinics. Inherited myths have ceased to provide limits for action. If the species is to survive the loss of its traditional myths, it must learn to cope rationally and politically with its envious, greedy and lazy dreams. Politically established limits to industrial growth will have to take the place of mythological boundaries. Political exploration and recognition of the necessary material conditions for equity and effectiveness will have to set limits to the industrial mode of production.

Endemic Nemesis

Nemesis has become structural and endemic. Increasingly manmade misery is the by-product of enterprises that were supposed to protect the ordinary people in their struggle with the inclemency of the environment and against the wanton injustice inflicted on them by the élite. The main source of pain, of disability and of death, has become engineered, albeit non-intentional, harassment. Our prevailing ailments, helplessness and injustice are largely the side-effects of strategies for more and better education, housing, diet or health.

A society which values planned teaching above autonomous learning cannot but teach man to keep to his engineered place. A society which relies for locomotion overwhelmingly on managed transport must do the same. Beyond a certain level of energy used for the acceleration of any one person in traffic, the transportation industry immobilizes and enslaves the majority of nameless passengers and provides advantages only to the élite. No new fuel, technology or public controls can keep the rising mobilization and acceleration of society from producing rising harriedness, programmed paralysis and inequality. The same is true for agriculture. Beyond a certain level of capital investment in the growing and processing of food, malnutrition must become pervasive.[251] The progress of the green revolution

[251] TEUTEBERG, Hans J., WIEGELMANN, Günter. *Der Wandel der Nahrungsgewohnheiten unter dem Einfluss der Industrialisierung.* Göttingen, Vandenhoeck & Ruprecht, 1972. Teuteberg and Wiegelmann assemble detailed history of the impact of industrialization on nutritional habits. The military needs of an emerging nationstate transformed the concern for food production and for well nourished recruits into an affair of state. Throughout antiquity and the Middle Ages the observance of dietetic rules was considered the principal discipline necessary to maintain health and extend a healthy life. HEISCHKEL-ARTELT, Edith. *Grundzüge der menschlichen Ernährung im Altertum und Mittelalter,* in: Proceedings of the 7th International Congress of Nutrition. Hamburg, 1966, Vol. 4. Braunschweig, 1967. This comparison of hundreds of cookery books from all ages indicates that health maintenance rather than taste was the primary concern of the rationally designed menu. Most of the food eaten by the inhabitants of European cities before the French Revolution was produced in the immediate neighbourhood. It was grown in fields from where it

must then rack the livers of consumers more effectively than Zeus's vulture. No biological engineering can prevent under-nourishment and food poisoning beyond this point. What is happening in the sub-Saharan Sahel is only a dress rehearsal for the encroaching world famine. This is but the application of a general law. When more than a certain proportion of value is produced by the industrial mode, subsistence activities are paralysed, equity declines and the total satisfaction in that particular area diminishes. In other words, beyond a certain level of industrial hubris, Nemesis *must* set in.

The lack of public attention to the imminence of famine is impressive. 1972 was the first year since World War II in which production of fish, an important source of animal feed, fertilizers and human food, declined, despite the increased capital and operational outlays of the fishing industry. Per capita production of agricultural products has fallen in developing countries to 1961–1965 levels, that is, to levels which had been reached before the peak of the 'green revolution'. In these countries, the market-able production of food has ceased to keep up with population increases, while during the past fifteen years many more people have moved out of the subsistence sector and have become dependent on the market. It is the first occasion in peacetime in which major stocks for the world market in grain have become

---

could be transported to city markets within a few hours, or it was grown in back yards. The multiple city ordinances limiting pigs and fowl on public streets reflected the ability of the city to produce part of its own food. Very few people could choose the kind of food they were going to eat, and unusual foods were considered un-healthy. Pre-industrial levels of nutrition in rural areas varied with the weather. With industrialization, urban nutrition became increasingly worse. Rural hunger changed from periodic inescapable destiny to a technically and financially manipul-able event. The need for workers to be well nourished in order to be productive was discovered around the middle of the 19th century. The need for public concern with their nutrition was discovered almost at the same time at which school-ing and medical care were first related to their productivity. By 1860 the need for good infant feeding was formally recognized by the German military. By that time the new kind of industrial undernourishment had already had its effects, and up to 40% of recruits had to be rejected. See HELLWING. *Über die Abnahme der Kriegstüchtigkeit in der Mark Brandenburg*, in: Mittheilungen des Kgl. Preussischen Statistischen Bureaus 1860, Nr. 9, 10 und 16. See also ABEL, Wilhelm. *Agrarkrisen und Agrarkon-junktur. Eine Geschichte der Land- und Ernahrungswirtschaft Mitteleuropas seit dem hohen Mittelalter*. 2. Aufl. Hamburg/Berlin, 1966. MARSHALL, C. *Health and nutri-tional consequences of selected developmental programmes*. This is section 1 in FARVAR, T. *The careless technology*. National History Press, N.J., 1972.

depleted. For the first time since railroads have made a true world-market in food possible, the world's population depends on current production, in other words, on weather and politics.

In former times, when hit by food shortages, people competed simply by force of their numbers for scarce foods. Affluence has now precipitated a brutal new competition between meat eaters and grain eaters. To feed an American, a ton of grain a year is needed, of which he eats only 150 lbs. in the form of cereals, while the rest is fed to livestock which give him eggs, meat and milk. A Mexican peasant will eat well, *and* feed his chickens, if he can get hold of 320 lbs. of grain per year. The political detente between major powers only sharpens this competition. It has depleted American food stocks, raised world prices, and fed enough Russian hogs to help the Kremlin proceed on its way to consumer-socialism.

As in 1973 with fuel, so it will be in 1976 with proteins: the world is turning from a buyer's into a seller's market. The fuel and food crises converge. Each pound of fertilizer requires from 5 to 10 pounds of fossil fuel to make and transport. Rising fuel prices decrease the amount of water people can pump. Much of the recently increased cost of food production has been due to increased costs of pumping and the use of large amounts of expensive fertilizers. The time the green revolution[252] could perhaps have bought for the spread and acceptance of birth control measures has run out. Hunger now controls population growth. But it is a new kind. It will not be the sporadic famine which formerly came with droughts and wars,[253] or the occasional food shortage that could be remedied by goodwill and emergency shipments. The coming hunger is a by-product of the inevitable concentration of industrialized agriculture in rich countries and in the fertile regions of poor countries. Paradoxically, the attempt to counter famine by further increases in industrially efficient agriculture only widens the scope of the catastrophe by depress-

---

[252] BORGSTROM, George. *The green revolution*, in: Focal Points, MacMillan, 1973, part II, pp. 172–201. Reproduced in CIDOC DOC I/V 74/67. This is an analysis and appraisal of a dozen illusions about the green revolution, many of which are constantly reinforced by misleading statements from international agencies.

[253] LEBRUN, François. *Les hommes et la mort en Anjou aux 17e et 18 siècles*, Essai de démographie et de psychologie historiques. Paris, Mouton, 1971. A detailed sociological-historical study.

ing the use of marginal lands. Famine will increase until the trend towards capital intensive food production by the poor for the rich has been replaced by a new kind of labour-intensive, regional, rural autonomy.[254]

Defenders of industrial progress are either blind or corrupt if they pretend that they can calculate the price of progress. The torts resulting from Nemesis cannot be compensated, calculated or liquidated.[255] The down-payment for industrial development

[254] HEIERLI, Urs. *Energiekrise und Entwicklungsstrategie. Dezentralisierte Entwicklung als Konsequenz der Energieverknappung*, 1974, 38 pp. mimeo.

[255] The imminent world crisis due to a new kind of malnutrition has at least four distinct contributing factors. The first is a simple decline in the quantity of food-stuffs available everywhere and the concentration of animal proteins on a minority of the world's population. The rich monopolize the sun's energy, so to speak, on their dinner tables. The second factor is the increase of unhealthy food additives which range from the remnants of pesticides, fungicides, or growth-promoting agents that the farmer delivers to the wholesaler, all the way to the colorants, preservatives and other by-products of packaging that the modern market requires. A third factor is the increase in mycotoxins, see TAINSH, Ramsay A. *Secondary mycotoxicosis*, 10 pp, Nov. 22, 1973, CIDOC, the poisons produced by fungi that inevitably grow when cereals and oil kernels are preserved over long periods or transported through different climates. The fourth factor is a growing cultural, genetic and physiological disparity between the food offered for consumption and the consumer.

The increase in mycotoxins, the third factor mentioned above, has been studied by our colleague Arturo ALDAMA in CIDOC at Cuernavaca. If his fears about the prevalence and gravity of mycotoxicosis are substantiated, the dangers to mankind from this source are greater than from rising radiation levels.

Secondary mycotoxicosis was not a very general problem as long as people were not fed via a world market. Less than 1% of the total weight of food consumed by humanity came from outside their own region. Only after World War II did a majority of people come to depend for an increasing percentage of their total food intake on goods that had been marketed beyond their neighbourhood. This relatively new situation guarantees that most goods, and especially the grains that constitute the basis of nutrition for the poor, have been stored for long periods and transported through many climates. Under these conditions food is exposed to a high probability of multiple fungal infection. Sporulae produce mycotoxins, which, once formed, cannot be removed by any cleaning process, and eventually pass into the animal and human food chain. The world market in food guarantees an almost instant spread of any new fungus. Sub-lethal doses of mycotoxins are difficult to trace. If they could be, much of the food now marketed would have to be condemned. Mycotoxins seem to be cumulative poisons that begin by interfering with the functioning of brain cells and proceed to other vital organs. One proven effect of secondary mycotoxicosis is a lowered ability to digest, leading to a higher food intake on the part of those who suffer from sub-lethal fungus poisoning. A sudden decline of world population is one of the foreseeable results of rising mycotoxicosis. It is not unreasonable to assume that this was the mechanism which suddenly wiped out many neolithic populations. The Latin American highlands are studded with large culture centres which were abandoned in the course of one generation.

might fit on the label, but the compound interest instalments on expanding production now accrue in suffering that exceeds any notion of measure or price. Not even ransom would be a fitting term, because instead of release, payment brings further bondage.

At some point in the expansion of institutions 'homo economicus', driven by the pursuit of marginal benefits, turns into 'homo religiosus' sacrificing himself for industrial ideology. This happens when members of a society are regularly asked to pay an even higher price for industrially defined necessities in spite of evidence that they are purchasing more suffering with each unit. At this point, social behaviour begins to parallel that of the drug addict. Expectations become irrational and nightmarish. The self-inflicted portion of suffering outweighs the damages done by nature, and all the torts inflicted by neighbour. Hubris motivates self-destructive mass behaviour. Classical Nemesis was the punishment for the rash abuse of privilege. Industrialized nemesis is the retribution for dutiful participation in the pursuit of dreams unchecked by traditional mythology or new reasonable self-restraint.

War and hunger, pestilence and natural catastrophes, torture and madness remain man's companions, but they are now shaped into a new Gestalt by the nemesis that overreaches them. The greater the economic progress of any community, the greater the part played by industrial nemesis in pain, impairment, discrimination and death. The more intense the reliance on techniques making for dependence, the higher the rate of waste, degradation and pathogenesis which must be countered by yet other techniques and the larger the work force active in the removal of garbage, in the management of waste, and in the treatment of people who have been made redundant by progress. The disciplined study of Nemesis can provide the framework for understanding the growth of activities concerned with defence against the unwanted by-products of industrially motivated values. It ought to be the key field of research for those who are concerned with health care, healing and consoling.

Medical Nemesis

Tantalus was a king whom the gods invited to Olympus to share their meal. He purloined Ambrosia, the divine potion which gave the gods unending life. For punishment, he was made immortal—in Hades; and condemned to suffer unending hunger and thirst. When he bends down towards the river in which he stands the water recedes, and when he reaches for the fruit above his head the branches move out of his reach. Ethologists might say that medical nemesis has programmed him for compulsory counter-intuitive behaviour.

Craving for Ambrosia has now spread to the common mortal. Scientific and political euphoria have combined to propagate the addiction. To sustain it a priesthood of Tantalus has organized itself, offering unlimited medical improvement in human health. The members of this guild pass themselves off as disciples of healing Aesculapius, while in fact they are pedlars of Ambrosia. The result of dependence on Ambrosia is Medical Nemesis.

Medical Nemesis is more than all clinical iatrogeneses put together, more than the sum of malpractice, negligence, professional callousness, political maldistribution, medically decreed disability and all the consequences of medical trial and error. It is the expropriation of man's coping ability by a maintenance service which keeps him geared up at the service of the industrial system.

Clinical iatrogenesis can be conceived of as a tort which calls for an indictment of doctors, pharmacists, hospitals and planners. Social iatrogenesis can at least be partially attributed to the prevalence of private over public interests governing the health professions. Structural iatrogenesis knows no defendant against whom a complaint can be lodged. It is spawned by a cancerous delusion about life, and manifests itself when this delusion has pervaded a culture. It is a symptom of the mortal sickness of medical civilization. No matter how thoroughly the medical-industrial complex is controlled or even curtailed, this limitation on one major industry cannot stem industrial nemesis. It would only transfer the social control now performed by medicine to some other hegemony. Only the inversion of society's overall growth rate in marketed goods and services can permit a reversal. But this does not make the medical profession a less crucial target for radical disestablishment: if a political consensus were reached that the outputs of the medical industry can be drastically reduced and that this can be done in the interests of better health, a major step would be taken to recognize the need for analogous reversals in other major industrial sectors. And since medicine is a sacred cow, its slaughter would have a 'vibration effect': people who can face suffering and death without need for magicians and mystagogues are free to rebel against other forms of expropriation now practised by teachers, engineers, lawyers, priests and party officials.

Veiled Nemesis

Industrial Nemesis in its various forms is now so prevalent that it is mistakenly assumed always to have been an integral part of the human condition. This trivialization of nemesis leads to a desperate inability to envisage its industrial origin and to seek its reversal in a negative growth of the industrial and managerial system which keeps us in its shackles.

Reactions to impending disaster still take the form of better educational curricula, more health-maintenance services or more efficient and less polluting energy transformers. The answer to nemesis is still sought in better engineering of industrial systems. The syndrome corresponding to nemesis is recognized, but its aetiology is still sought in bad engineering compounded by self-serving management whether under the control of Wall Street or of The Party. Nemesis is not yet recognized to be the materialization of a social answer to a greedy, envious and lazy dream. Nemesis is not yet understood to be the ranting delusion fostered by the non-technical, ritual structure of our major industrial institutions. Just as Galileo's contemporaries refused to look through the telescope at Jupiter's moons because they feared that their heliocentric world-view would be shaken, so our contemporaries refuse to face nemesis because they feel incapable of putting the autonomous rather than the industrial mode of production at the centre of their socio-political constructs.

From Inherited Myth to Respectful Procedure

Among primitives and throughout recorded history the power of a symbolic dimension has always been recognized; people saw themselves as being threatened by the tremendous, the awesome, the fey. This dimension not only set boundaries to the power of the king and the magician, but also to that of the artisan and the technician. Indeed, Malinowski claims that no society other than ours has allowed the use of available tools to their utmost efficiency. Until now, recognizing a sacred dimension was a necessary foundation for ethics.[256] After several generations of oblivion, the finiteness of nature intrudes again upon our consciousness. I argue that at this moment of crisis it would be a grave mistake to found the limit of human actions on some substantive ecological ideology which would modernize the mythic sacredness of nature. Only a widespread agreement on the procedures through which the autonomy of post-industrial man can be equitably guaranteed will lead to the recognition of the necessary limits to human action.

In a world in which engineering provides the norms, human action is turned into something other than it had naturally been. Common to all ethics was the assumption that the human act is performed within the human condition. Since the various ethical systems assumed, tacitly or explicitly, that this human condition was more or less given, once and for all, the range of human action was narrowly circumscribed. Nature was considered more or less invulnerable: if its boundaries were transgressed, it took vengeance on the transgressor, be he Icarus, Oedipus, Prometheus or even Xerxes. A clear distinction reigned between tools that had been given to mankind by the gods and that worked within the harmony of a cosmic nexus and other types of machines like the wings made by Icarus to outwit the wisdom of this nexus of forces. 'Techne'—the art that produced the first type of tool—was a measured tribute to necessity and not the road to mankind's chosen action. Men and women faced gods to whom they attributed purpose, thereby perceiving the intentionality of their own action as circumscribed and given meaning by intentions of a higher order.

In our industrialized epoch, however, not only the object, but also the very nature of human action is new. Instead of facing gods who act we confront the blind forces of nature, and instead of facing the dynamic limits of a universe which we have now

---

[256] JONAS, Hans. *Technology and responsibility: reflections on the new task of ethics*, in: Social Research, 1972, pp. 31–54.

come to know, we act as if these limits did not translate into critical thresholds for human action. Traditionally the categorical imperative could circumscribe and validate action as being truly human; directly enjoining limits to one's actions, it demanded respect for the equal freedom of others. Indirectly this imperative recognized limits to action set by the human condition. The loss of a normative 'human condition' not only introduces a newness into the human act, but also a newness into the human attitude towards the framework in which a person acts. If this action is to remain human after the framework has been deprived of its sacred character, it needs a recognized ethical foundation within a new type of imperative. This imperative can be summed up only as follows: 'act so that the effect of your action is compatible with the permanence of genuine human life'; very concretely applied this could mean: 'do not raise radiation levels unless you know that this action will not be visited on your grandchild'. Such an imperative obviously cannot be formulated as long as 'genuine human life' is considered an infinitely elastic concept.

Is it possible, without restoring the category of the sacred, to attain the ethics that alone would enable mankind to accept the extreme discipline of this new imperative? If not, rationalizations would have to be forthcoming for any atrocity: 'why should background radiation not be raised? Our grandchildren will get used to it!' In some instances, fear might help preserve minimal sanity, but only when there are consequences that are fairly imminent. Breeder-reactors might not become operational for fear that they may serve the Mafia for next year's extortions or cause cancer before the operator dies, but only the awe of the sacred, with its unqualified veto, has so far proven independent of the computations of mundane self-interest and the solace of uncertainty about remote consequences, and this could now be re-evoked as stringent enough to impose the imperative which says that genuine human life deserves respect both now and in the future.[257] In fact, this recourse to the sacred has been blocked

[257] RAMSEY, Paul. *Fabricated man: the ethics of genetic control.* New Haven, Yale Univ. Press, 1970. There are things that we can do, and that ought not to be done. To exclude these things is a necessary condition for saving man from total abasement by technology.

in our present crisis. Recourse to faith could provide an escape for those who believe, but it cannot found an ethical imperative, because faith is either there or not there; and if it is absent, the faithful cannot blame the infidel. Recent history has shown that the taboos of traditional cultures are irrelevant in combating an over-extension of industrial production. After all, the effectiveness of these taboos had been tied to the values of a particular society and its mode of production, and it is precisely these that have been irrevocably lost in the process of industrialization. It is not necessary, probably not feasible, and certainly not desirable, to base the limitation of industrial societies on a shared system of substantive beliefs which would have to be enforced by police power aiming at the common good. It is possible to find the needed basis for ethical human action without depending on the shared recognition of any ecological dogmatism now in vogue. This alternative to a new ecological religion or ideology is based on an agreement about basic values and on procedural rules.

It can be demonstrated that, beyond a certain point in the expansion of industrial production in any major field of value, the marginal utilities must cease to be equitably distributed and that, simultaneously, overall effectiveness begins to decline. If the industrial mode of production expands beyond a certain stage and continues to impinge on the autonomous mode, increasing personal suffering and social dissolution set in. In the interim, that is, between the point of optimal synergy between industrial and autonomous production and the point of maximum tolerable industrial hegemony, political and juridical procedures become necessary to reverse industrial expansion. If these procedures are conducted in a spirit of enlightened self-interest and a desire for survival and with equitable distribution of social outputs and equitable access to social control, the outcome ought to be a recognition of the carrying capacity of the environment and of the optimal industrial complement to autonomous action needed for the effective pursuit of personal goals. Political procedures orientated to the value of survival in distributive and participatory equity is the only rational answer to increasing total management in the shadow of ecological ideology.

The recovery of personal autonomy will thus be the result of political action reinforcing an ethical awakening. People will want to limit transportation, because they will want to move efficiently, freely and with equity; they will limit education, because they will want to share equally the opportunity, time and interest to learn *in* rather than *about* the world; people will limit medical therapies because they will want to conserve their opportunity and power to heal. They will recognize that only the disciplined limitation of power can provide equitably shared satisfaction.

The recovery of autonomous action will depend not on new specific goals people share, but on their use of legal and political procedures that permit individuals and groups to resolve conflicts arising from their pursuit of different goals. Better mobility will not depend on some new kind of transportation system, but on conditions which make personal mobility under personal control more valuable. Better learning opportunities will not depend on more information about the world better distributed, but on the limitation of capital intensive production for the sake of interesting working conditions. Better health care will not depend on some new therapeutic standard, but on the level of willingness and competence to engage in self-care. The recovery of this power depends on the recognition of our present delusions.

The Right to Health

Increasing and irreparable damage accompanies present industrial expansion in all sectors. In medicine these damages appear as iatrogenesis. Iatrogenesis is clinical when pain, sickness and death result from medical care; it is social when health policies reinforce an industrial organization which generates ill health; it is structural when medically sponsored behaviour and delusions restrict the vital autonomy of people by undermining their competence in growing up, caring for each other and aging, or when medical intervention disables personal responses to pain, disability, impairment, anguish and death.

Most of the remedies now proposed by the social engineers and economists to reduce iatrogenesis include a further increase of medical controls. These so-called remedies generate second-order iatrogenic ills on each of the three critical levels.

The most profound iatrogenic effects of the medical techno-structure are a result of its non-technical functions, by which it supports the increasing institutionalization of values. The technical and the non-technical consequences of institutional medicine coalesce and generate a new kind of suffering: anaesthetized, impotent and solitary survival in a world turned into a hospital ward. Medical nemesis is the experience of people who are largely deprived of any autonomous ability to cope with nature, neighbour and dreams, and who are technically maintained within environmental, social and symbolic systems. Medical nemesis cannot be measured, but its experience can be shared. The intensity with which it is experienced will depend on the independence, vitality and relatedness of each individual.

The perception of nemesis leads to a choice. Either the natural boundaries of human endeavour are estimated, recognized and translated into politically determined limits, or the alternative to extinction is accepted as compulsory survival in a planned and engineered hell. Until recently the choice between the politics of voluntary poverty and the hell of the systems engineer did not fit into the language of scientists or politicians. Our increasing experience with Medical Nemesis lends new significance to the alternative: society must either choose the same stringent limits within which all its members find a guarantee for equal freedom, or it will have to accept unprecedented hierarchical controls.

In several nations the public is now ready for a review of its health care system. There is a serious danger that the forthcoming debate will reinforce the present frustrating medicalization of life and thereby heighten Nemesis.

The debate could still be rescued if attention were focused on Medical Nemesis, if recuperation of personal responsibility for health-care were made the central issue, and if limitations on professional monopolies were made the major goal of legislation. Instead of limiting the resources of doctors and of the institutions that employ them, such legislation would proscribe medical technology to professionals until those devices and means that can be handled by laymen are truly available to anyone wanting access to them. Instead of multiplying the specialists who can grant any one of the variety of sick-roles to people who are made ill by their work and their life, the new legislation would guarantee the right of people to drop out and to organize for a less destructive way of life, in which they would have more con-

166

trol of their environment. Instead of restricting access to addictive, dangerous or useless drugs and procedures, such legislation would shift the full burden of their responsible use to the sick man and his next of kin. Instead of submitting the physical and mental integrity of citizens to more and more wardens, such legislation would recognize each man's right to define his own health—subject only to limitations imposed by respect for his neighbour's rights. Instead of relying on professional expertise to verify such values that will guide them. Instead of strengthening the licensing power of specialized peers and government agencies, new legislation would allow popular choice to entitle elected healers to tax-supported health jobs. Instead of submitting their performance to professional review organizations, new legislation would have them evaluated by the community they serve. Such guarantees against the medical support of a sickening industrial system would set the stage for the practice of health as a virtue.

Hygiene as a Virtue

Health designates a process of adaptation. It is not the result of instinct, but of an autonomous yet culturally shaped reaction to socially created reality. It designates the ability to adapt to changing environments, to growing up and to aging, to healing when damaged, to suffering and to the peaceful expectation of death. Health embraces the future as well, and therefore includes anguish and the inner resources to live with it.[258]

Health designates a process by which each is responsible, but only in part responsible to others. To be responsible may mean two things. A man is responsible for what he has done, and responsible to another person or group. Only when he feels subjectively responsible or answerable to another person will the consequences of his failure be not reprehension, criticism, censure or punishment, but regret, remorse and true repentance. The consequent states of grief and distress are marks of recovery and healing, and are phenomenologically something entirely different from the guilt feelings usually described in psychoanalytic

[258] BERGER, Peter. *The social construction of reality: a treatise on the sociology of knowledge*, N.Y., Doubleday, 1966.

literature. Health is a task, and as such not comparable to the physiological balance of beasts. Success in this personal task is in large part the result of the self-awareness, self-discipline and inner resources by which each person regulates his own daily rhythm and actions, his diet and his sex. Knowledge encompassing desirable activities, competent performance, commitment to enhance health in others—these are all learned through example from peers or elders. These personal activities are shaped and conditioned by the culture in which the individual grows up: patterns of work and leisure, of celebration and of sleep, of production and preparation of food and drink, of family patterns and politics. The existence of long-tested health patterns which fit a geographic area and a technical situation depend to a large extent on long-lasting political autonomy. They depend on the spread of responsibility for healthy habits and for the socio-biological environment. That is, they depend on the dynamic stability of a culture.

Traditionally, cultures were concerned primarily with the health of their members. As cultures set themselves other goals, health care became a privilege for an élite. The building of a pyramid, the conquest of the Holy Land, or the landing on the moon are equally distracting from the health-sustaining integrity of a social system. The need for specialized, professional health care beyond a certain point can be taken as an indication of the unhealthy goals pursued by society. Where the identity of culture and health maintenance have succumbed to a civilization structurally orientated towards unlimited progress, the maintenance of health becomes increasingly a matter of virtue, that is, of consciously formed habit. To be healthy becomes an enlightened task. It also turns into an anti-social activity. An unhealthy society depends on unhealthy people whose survival, discipline and functioning are assured through delivery of the necessary therapeutic services.

The level of public health corresponds to the degree to which the means and responsibility for coping with illness are distributed amongst the total population. This ability to cope can be enhanced but never replaced by medical intervention in the lives of people or by the hygienic characteristics of the environment. That society which can reduce professional intervention to the minimum will provide the best conditions for health. The greater the potential for autonomous adaptation to self, to others and to the environment, the less management of adaptation will be needed or tolerated.

A world of optimal and widespread health is obviously a world of minimal and only occasional medical intervention. Healthy people are those who live in healthy homes on a healthy diet; in an environment equally fit for birth, growth, work, healing and dying: sustained by a culture which enhances the conscious acceptance of limits to population, of aging, of incomplete recovery and ever imminent death. Healthy people need no bureaucratic interference to mate, give birth, share the human condition and die.

Man's consciously lived fragility, individuality and relatedness make the experience of pain, of sickness and of death an integral part of his life. The ability to cope with this trio autonomously is fundamental to his health. As he becomes dependent on the management of his intimacy, he renounces his autonomy and his health *must* decline. The true miracle of modern medicine is diabolical. It consists not only of making individuals but whole populations survive on inhumanly low levels of personal health. That health should decline with increasing health service delivery is unforeseen only by the health managers, precisely because their strategies are the result of their blindness to the inalienability of life.

BIBLIOGRAPHICAL INDEX

This bibliographical index contains all the authors and titles of books or articles referred to in the footnotes. Though many of the footnotes list a large number of publications, the publishers have decided to provide page references only, rather than including the footnote number as well.

177

179